DOIN ONE
FOR THE TEAM
YEARS IN THE SWINGING LIFESTYLE

Simbaxxx

BookSurge, LLC
North Charleston, South Carolina

Publisher: BookSurge, LLC
North Charleston, South Carolina
www.booksurge.com
1-866-308-6235
orders@booksurge.com

To My Husband

- My best friend and soul mate

♥ ♥ ♥

THE SIX MISTAKES OF MAN

- The illusion that personal gain is made up of crushing others.

- The tendency to worry about things that cannot be changed or corrected.

- Insisting that a thing is impossible because we cannot accomplish it.

- Refusing to set aside trivial preferences.

- Neglecting development and refinement of the mind and not acquiring the habit of reading and study.

- Attempting to compel others to believe and live as we do.

MARCUS TULLIUS CICERO
(106 B.C. – 43 B.C.)
ROMAN STATESMAN AND PHILOSOPHER

CONTENTS

LOVE'S PHILOSOPHY

I
The fountains mingle with the river
And the rivers with the Ocean,
The winds of Heaven mix forever
With a sweet emotion;
Nothing in the world is single;
All things by a law divine
In one spirit meet and mingle.
Why not I with thine?

See the mountains kiss high Heaven
And the waves clasp one another;
No sister-flower would be forgiven
If it distained its' brother;
And the sunlight clasps the earth
And the moonbeams kiss the sea;
What is all this sweet work worth
if thou kiss not me?

PERCY BYSSHE SHELLEY
(1792-1822)
English philosophical poet

Introduction

Your neighbors are doing the horizontal cha-cha with other couples and you don't even know it. Most of you are clueless to the erotic activities that are right under your nose. I could even be one of your neighbors!

The white picket fenced neighborhoods are laced with carnal desires and this once thought extinct, "wife swapping" has exploded into a rapidly growing commercial industry and a way of life for the common Joe and Mary. I know, because my husband and I have been swingers for 3 years now. My Ms. Accountant attitude by day has everyone fooled. There are a lot of misconceptions about Swingers and I am the first to admit that I, too, had many stereotyped opinions of Swingers, prior to delving deeper in to this erotic Lifestyle.

First off, discard the thinking that people in the Lifestyle have troubled marriages and are somehow reflecting unhealthy personality disorders. I am here to tell you that your doctor, lawyer, banker, mortgage broker, stock broker, dentist, financial advisor, teacher, mother (yes, I said your mother), nurse and best golf buddy could be keeping a big secret from you. If you find deep compassion for others, loyal friendships, spiritually rich values and unconditional love for your spouse all odd, then you definitely don't want to become a Swinger, because it's those types of fine qualities in people that you'll find in the Lifestyle. The funny part about it, once we decided to investigate swinging we had no idea how prevalent it was in main stream suburbia. They are everywhere - holding parties' right under your nose. Did you ever wonder why mom and dad had these unusually close friends and seemed to go to a lot of long movies? Movies my ass! They were heading for a swing party. You think I'm kidding? How about that neighbor down the street that throws those once a month parties (that you never get invited to) where the people only arrive after dark and all the women are wearing high heels (of course, fuck me pumps). I'm telling you right now, it's much more prevalent than you ever suspect. By the time you finish this book you are going to question if certain friends of yours (and relatives) are really Swingers. I would bet you know one and you just aren't aware of it.

I'll never forget the first time my boyfriend (now husband) asked me if I wanted to observe something different and go to a swing club. I actually thought he was kidding and I laughingly made the remark, "Didn't that go out in the 50's before I was born?" I was shocked that it was still around and flourishing. He gave me a weeks' warning and promised all we had to do was just observe. That entire week I was very excited about the possibilities but also stressed regarding the unknown. I had no idea what to expect and wondered if I would have to beat peoples' advances off and their attempts to touch me. The party was up in the hills of Malibu and driving up the coast road that night I was very quiet. The top was down on our car and the beautiful stars were glowing but all I could do was think about what I was getting into that evening. We had only been dating for about three weeks and I was feeling some very confusing and conflicting ideas about the evenings' possibilities. I had to put total confidence in to him to control this new situation, because I was feeling totally out of control of not knowing the guidelines of such a foreign Lifestyle. Although, my husband had never attended a swing club either, it somehow didn't bother him like the all consuming internal dialog that I was having with myself. As we wound up the road towards the estate there were many things spinning through my mind. Was I wearing the right outfit? How would people react to us? Would people approach us? What *if* people approached us? Are people walking around naked? Is it a free-for all with people grabbing anyone they can find and playing with them? What if I told someone "No" and they wouldn't take "No" as my answer? Would people be pushy and grab at me? What was expected of me? Needless to say, my mind was in the carpool lane.

My thoughts were racing so fast that I noticed nothing but my preoccupation of the unknown as the car approached the club.

I learned a lot that first night and the past three years in the Lifestyle I have also learned every facet of swinging; but more importantly I learned a lot about myself, other people and normal human nature. I went in wanting to just dabble in carnal desires but came out of my experiences having learned much more.

Chapter One

CARNAL
DESIRES

The Lifestyle is based on a traditional emotional monogamy relationship, flavored with eroticism of sexual non-monogamy.

Couples in the Lifestyle know me as Simbaxxx. I'm a married working mother, putting in forty hours a week in the very conservative world of accounting. I grew up in the Midwest, in a traditional household with loving parents and a father that was even a minister. I know you must be questioning the fact that I was raised with spiritual values, yet participate in the swing Lifestyle? How could I possibly fit the two together? Very easily, once I got past the misconceptions that the vanilla world (non-swingers) seems to manufacturer for this popular, but misunderstood Lifestyle.

Growing up, I was never a person to accept anything just because it's the "norm" or just because it was traditional. I have always thought each individual needs to search in their own heart what makes sense to them, instead of just blindly following the herd. I was that girl in the church confirmation class that raised her hand to question a few of those initial inconsistencies I spotted in traditional doctrines. Let's see, I believe it went something like this....

Simba: *"Now let me get this straight. You are saying God is everywhere?"*

Teacher: *"Yes, that is correct. God is everywhere and sees all."*

Simba: *"Okay......so, if he is everywhere, that means he is inside me."*

Teacher: *"Aaah, well aaaah......"*

Simba: *"Wait a minute. You just said he was everywhere and if that's correct then that means he is inside me and that means I am God and so are you, you and you. Is that what you are saying?"*

Teacher: *"No that is not what I'm saying."*

Simba: *"OH, I see! He is everywhere, but he isn't everywhere. Okaaaaay, now I've got it."*

I passed confirmation class with flying colors, but I think it was just because they didn't want me back for more dingbat questions. This was one of my first clues in life that I looked at things differently. "Why?" was my favorite word.

It took me years to get to the root of my conflicts with most traditional based thinking. In the end, it mostly came down to the fact that a lot of things seem to be governed by fear rather than love -

from structured religion to traditional relationships. My own heart told me life should be governed solely by love and compassion for others and not through fear and restrictions.

I lived in a marriage for 20 years made of traditional values and beliefs and although it's certainly fine for many, the fear based restrictions didn't fit my inner beliefs. If you love someone with the purest unconditional love, then you only want things that are happy and fulfilling for them. Unconditional love for your spouse, requires you to love them for who they are and not trying to change them to fit your needs. I think when the truth is out; most people in traditional relationships base their love on it being conditional. I love you IF you act this way or I love you IF you respond the way I think you should.

My first husband had fear based love for me and squeezed the love right out of my heart. The harder you try to hold onto something, the faster it will slip through your fingers. Those 20 years trying to conform to traditional values ended as many marriages in divorce. It was important for me to find a mate that would accept and love me as I am and the reverse for him from me. It took me 42 years to find him, but I finally met and married my soul mate, lover, best friend, buddy and boyfriend - all wrapped into one. Finally a relationship based on freedom and love instead of fear and restrictions.

When my husband and I met, we both had interest in sexual experimentation, while not wanting to jeopardize our relationship or affection for one another. We wanted an emotionally monogamous relationship where two individuals in love, could seek adventure together. We soon found that one of the immense enjoyments was to observe each other laughing and playing while engaged in recreational sexual activity with others, but saving our emotionally tender "love making" for only one another.

Just ponder the concept of sharing your mate openly with others. You might be surprised how this quiet sexual revolution is growing beyond its hidden boundaries. I know what you are thinking. "How could someone do that if they are in love?" "What about jealousy issues?" "Can people just observe others playing together and not actively participate at swing clubs?" "How do you find and meet people and what are the guidelines?" "What is the difference between soft swap and full swap?" "How could seeing your mate having sex with another person be a turn on?" "How do we go about exploring these avenues without jeopardizing our marriage or doing something that we might regret later?"

The Lifestyle is based on a traditional emotional monogamy relationship, flavored with eroticism of sexual non-monogamy. What was once labeled as "wife swapping" years ago, has modernized to the " Lifestyle" and expanded its' boundaries to encapsulate varying degrees of eroticism with millions of members and vast connected networks, mainstream resorts, organizations and legal "couples only" on-site sex play clubs through out the world. Go ahead! Just look up swing clubs on the internet and you'll be shocked at how prevalent they are in today's suburbia. They are no longer the couples of the 50's where the male was the center and catalyst for the swinging with the wife playing the subordinate role. The ease of communication and connection with people of similar interests through the internet has perpetuated the explosion of interest because of the autonomy. The big change of today's Lifestyle is the dominance and control by the females. They control a lot of the   aspects of the solicitation, meeting, boundaries and direction that the couple takes on their adventures together.

With society's present divorce rate still on the rise along, with infidelity, this Lifestyle is now becoming more commonplace with Baby Boomers and even the younger crowd. Those of you that are brave enough, start asking your friends if any of them have had   experiences in the past with group sexual activities or if they have thought about the subject. Most people have some interest, if only to find out the erotic details of what they may deem as a taboo.

So just what is normal human nature? I think if we were more honest with one another we would admit that even though we are compelled by erotic decadence, most people just don't like being classified outside of tradition (except for me…ha ha). Tradition is the safe zone where everyone is accepted and no one likes to rock the boat too much.   Let's face it, our erotic randy thoughts are always there and even we girls can come up with some of the most explicit sexual ideas, but in most cases we are too embarrassed to reveal it.   Women are raised with an emphasis on being a "good girl" which means she is to find her life partner and enjoy sex with only him the rest of her life. Men are raised to think that the more sexual experience they have the more masculine they are perceived.   The more playing around they can experience the more they are seen as a normal healthy male. With the changes in the 60's with the birth control pill and the more independent career woman arriving to the forefront, we have slowly over the decades become more acceptant of females participating in premarital sex without labeling them "slutty". The double standard is still out there but it seems to be lessening with time.

♥ ♥ ♥

It was on our very first date, when my husband-to-be asked if I had any interest in women or if I had ever thought of having sex in front of other people. I knew right then this guy was going to give me a rollercoaster ride and steal my heart in the process with his open attitude. He was 52 at the time and felt he could waste no time in dating someone that did have the same adventurous attitude. I did admit on that first date that I had touched another girl on one of those overnight slumber parties in the 6th grade and that having sex in front others certainly peaked my interest.

Remember back to your youthful years, when you were fascinated with how your genitals looked, but more importantly the huge impact of actually seeing someone else's privates. I'll never forget my two girlfriends and I at age eleven were spending the night at one of their homes and the topic of oral sex came up in our discussions. We were fascinated about what few details we had between us. I lifted my nightgown and flashed my privates to my girlfriends. I asked my girlfriend if I could see her privates and compare the differences. She lay back on the bed spreading her legs and I started touching her inner lips with my fingers. I found it fascinating that even though she had the same hardware, it was somehow different and that made it so interesting My girlfriend's body was beautiful just like mine and although I remembered the incident, I didn't repeat anything like it until college.

My husband-to-be was determined to help me "blossom" once he discovered our mutual admiration for the female body. I always found my own body interesting, beautiful and fun to play with, so naturally I wondered why people wouldn't think it such a stretch to enjoy other women's bodies that are exactly the same as my own. Our bodies are beautiful! No matter the shape, size or weight… they are damn erotic! The idea of pursuing this avenue, even though titillating, also scared the holy crap out me. Let's face it, up until this point, I was pretty sheltered. I didn't know whether to hug my husband-to-be or run as fast as I could! Needless to say, I ended up marrying him two years later after many wonderful swinging and non-swinging experiences. Swinging has never been at the forefront of our relationship, but just a small part of our life that added that extra zing to it.

♥ ♥ ♥

Men and women seem to view sex a bit different. Women seem to concentrate more on the romantic aspect of sex; whereas, the men ususaly concentrate on more of the physical side of sex. Women are taught from day one to pursue romantic sex! Otherwise, women have been targeted as a slut. It's the raw animalistic recreational sex and not romance that is usually sought after in swinging. Your spouse or partner provides you the emotional romantic loving sex, but it's the various other partners in the Lifestyle that give you that recreational sex.

The seeking of loving romantic sex versus the recreational sex hasn't changed much over the centuries. It just depends what century you happen to be born into for how prevalent sexual freedom is in society.

I believe the earliest writing of sex was around 3200BC in Mesopotamia. Men could have sex with other women, but the same was not allowed for women (isn't that just like men). It was a King's duty to have intercourse with all the priestess in the temple for a bountiful year. It was also apparently a culture that thought of sex as "spiritual healing".

We can be pompous and intellectual about our motivations with sex; but, when it comes down to it the body, mind and genetics drive our erotic undertones and as long as they are not damaging to others, then I see them as healthy. I believe that history has suggested that the more you repress sexuality the more mental obsessions and unhealthy phobic problems seem to pop up. Also, it depends on which era you lived as to whether something was deemed by society as accepted or not. Incest is an unthinkable crime in today's society, but if you lived in Egypt 5000 years ago it was an accepted practice for the king and queen to be brother and sister. They needed to keep the royal blood line pure. Obviously not the smartest thing to do based on biology, but society accepted this practice as the "norm". Even in the most recent of times, the straight-laced Victorian era soon pushed the pendulum to swing to the other end of the spectrum with the   erotic decadence of the 1920's and the sexually promiscuous Flapper.

♥ ♥ ♥

So why do committed couples with loving sex lives decide to experiment with swinging? Many couples after being together for several years are looking for extra thrills together. They want to be honest and loving with their spouse and explore new adventures hand in hand. Who could be better than to explore new things in life but with your best friend and buddy?   Unfortunately, society labels many of the non-traditional sexual avenues as taboo, including swinging.   Fortunately, this is slowly changing as more and more committed couples want to find safe avenues to experiment and live out their fantasies.

I remember one of my fantasies was to have sex with my husband and be observed by others and to walk around and observe other people having sex but not necessarily participate. Do you have any idea how erotic it is to be able to walk through a club in the safety of your spouse and see over one hundred people through out the facility in every position of sexual exchange? It is thrilling! Even today my husband at times has to remind me to close my mouth, because I'm completely mesmerized. Our first visit to a large club I was so turned on after 30 minutes of watching other people that I had to have my husband find a dark corner to ourselves and relieve some of the pent up pressure inside me! That, too, was a new exciting feeling!

Swinging is a safe environment for couples to explore their sexual urges together. So, let's take a look at what makes up the "Lifestyle".

.

Chapter Two

THE LIFESTYLE

A common guideline in the Lifestyle is for the two females to bond, so they feel comfortable sharing their husbands.

Just who are these people experimenting in new ways to stimulate and strengthen their committed relationships? They use to be the stereo typical white professionals, 35 years old and in the middle and upper middle class. Over the recent years, I am seeing an assortment of just about all ethnic groups, classes and ages. Most couples that talk about the possibilities of experimenting with sex do so after the spark in their sex has dulled at around the 5 to 7 year mark. They are still deeply in love and committed to one another but it takes a lot more to excite them than the once simple caress that would work in the past. These couples have solid emotionally loving relationships and are looking for adventure to experience together. Many people will make the assumption that members of the Lifestyle are extremely outgoing and liberal in their values. I have met more conservatives in this Lifestyle than you can imagine! You will find all types are in the Lifestyle. A perfect example is my own husband. He is very conservative and I am much more liberal. So, we are two totally different type of personalities; but, both are very comfortable and satisfied in the Lifestyle with its' different aspects.

Many times one or both partners have unusually high libidos or in many cases they want to live out some fantasies (before they get too old) that both find interesting and fun. You know the fantasies I'm talking about. Ladies, who is your hottest looking close girlfriend? The one girlfriend who you trust inside and out with all your inner secrets and may also be married to a hot guy. So, let's say you are talking one day with your girlfriend that you just don't think you give good blow jobs and your husband is constantly asking for them. Your girlfriend tells you that she has been told she gives great head! So, you ask your girlfriend to teach you how to give great head. She agrees and invites you to watch her demonstrate it on her own husband. In the meantime, her husband is about ready to wet his pants he is so excited at the possibilities! That's how it happens......two women trusting each other to the point of having some sexual fun together and the husbands reaping the benefits of the exchange. Nothing serious and only lighthearted laughs about a simple subject that many talk about - blow jobs! It's these simple fantasies that easily become reality when two partners start openly talking about what excites them. It may not even involve direct contact with another couple but simply the couple finding the thought of others watching them have sex in a public place to be erotic. There are many couples in the Lifestyle that go to the clubs to have sex with each other in a group setting and never have sex with others.

There are different levels of participation in the Lifestyle and they are generally categorized in to two simple types. Inside these two types are infinite levels customized by the couple with specific parameters unique to that couples' needs.

Soft Swap

Newbies in the Lifestyle generally enter with their tip toes and not their whole foot! Maybe I should clarify that statement... most men would stick their whole foot in but it's we women that are bashful and unsure of what we will accept. Generally, it's the men that come up with the idea of getting into the Lifestyle and it's the woman's decision on how much or how little involvement the couple is going to explore. Usually, the woman is shy and unsure of what to expect. Soft swap is where many women prefer to start and set the pace. This includes starting with just voyeurism and not allowing others to touch to them. It then expands to touch and eventually all oral aspects of sex including giving head and/or eating pussy. It's at this point that the female has to make a decision as to whether she is intrigued by other women's touch (bi-curious) or is uncomfortable with another woman's sexual touches (straight). Soft swap, to its' fullest extent is all sexual play, except penetration.

Men in the Lifestyle are generally straight and aren't nearly as open about being bi or bi-curious with other men. It's not the "norm" for the man to be bi; although, there are certainly exceptions to the rule, but they are just not as prevalent. Unfortunately, it's still a double standard in this area.

All these new concepts need to be discussed thoroughly by the couple well in advance of any potential playing. Each needs to agree on their limitations and stick to their agreement. In the beginning, everything is usually foreign and so unknown to the female that most likely all she will want to do the first time out is just be a "lookeelou". Many times she will have preconceived fears of orgies where the women are flung on the shoulder of strangers and taken off in a corner and raped.

Let's get back to that very first time my husband-to-be took me to the Malibu swing club. Nervous as I was, I couldn't discount the idea of being able to just walk around a club with naked people all around and watching people have sex as an erotic enticement. I didn't want to be pressured to perform on any level and I made him promise we could just be voyeurs (like I really stuck to that one once we arrived). I had not been to anything remotely similar, so I had no idea what to expect. Everyone could roam freely inside and out without worry from the neighbors. I was scared, nervous and excited all at once. Knowing that there was no pressure to do anything helped me to relax and enjoy the new experiences. Most standard rules include normal stuff like single men not allowed, men have to stay with their mates and cannot roam freely by themselves and the all important "No" means "No". There were several designated couples there that were the host couples that kept an eye on things and if you needed help or had a problem you could just go to them. We were shown around and taken to the locker room to store our stuff. There were plenty of clean towel, showers, restrooms (co-ed, of course) and the toiletry items included bucket loads of condoms everywhere. Everyone around me had erotic lingerie on or sexy street clothes. The playrooms were clean and large and as my husband and I roamed around we watched people playing in all capacities of sex. It was an overwhelming feeling for me to watch these naked people walking around and playing with one another. At first we kept our clothes on because I wasn't comfortable with undressing for any reason. I wanted to watch! As my husband fondled and groped me in front of the people in the room we saw 6 couples enter through the front door all about the same time with bags in hand. They were all in their mid 30's and greeted each other, obviously, knowing one another well. As they all talked about mundane daily topics such as current events they proceeded to all undress. They all got naked and started playing. The women were playing with the women and then moved to the other men and after about an hour and a half (once every guy had banged all the other women in their little group) they all got dressed at the same time, kissed each other good-bye and left (I'm sure to relieve their babysitters).

We eventually found a couple open to play with us with just soft swapping in mind (you have to forewarn them you are soft swap or they will assume you are full swap). I played with the female and caressed and suckled her breasts and eventually went down on her. In the meantime, the men were caressing us and stroking themselves. My husband then went down on the other woman and I allowed her spouse to go down on me. Okay, I was hooked. It was exciting and scary; however, it was not scary enough to deter me from playing again with several couples over the next year.

We found it more difficult to find soft swap couples to play with because most people get into the Lifestyle for full swap. You also find that many experienced couples don't have the patience for Newbies because it can be frustrating to be with someone that doesn't know what they will or will not do since they are new to the whole experience. In the beginning, it can be hard to get started in a club unless you are going there to specifically meet someone. We never had problems going cold turkey not knowing anyone in the club and as we saw people playing and I would ask if I could caress the female. Then you just wait for a reaction. She will make it obvious if she wants you to touch her.

After about a year, we decided to full swap, but not without a lot of discussion on it for months prior to it ever happening.

Full Swap

Transitioning from soft swap to full swap can be a very big event. I think it can be a bigger decision for the female because innately it could be potentially more physically or psychologically more harmful. Nevertheless, I won't discount the man's own issues either when seeing another man pleasuring his wife who may or may not have ever been with another man. There can be a lot of issues going on in his head about these new set of events which we will discuss later. It can be an extremely confusing time also because the man (and the woman) are excited when another person touches and plays with them and yet apprehensive about watching their spouse perform and enjoy the touch of others. You have to take each step slow over many play sessions and after each experience, you must talk about what bothered you and what excited you both. It may take several months of making the transition. Some couples may only feel liking doing soft swap and others may venture further to full swap. Obviously you are not obligated to be full swap with every couple that you play with. To this day, we don't full swap with every couple. When making this transition, it's done with both spouses making this move to intercourse and uncommon for just one spouse to stay solely as soft swap. You are a team and should pursue new avenues together. Men, especially need to remember you are a team and you don't leave your wife in the dust by pursing intercourse while she doesn't want to make the same commitment to the Lifestyle. You hang back with her giving her emotional support that you are there for her and that she is number one in you life. You don't have to have full swap to have fun. If she senses even an ounce of disappointment on your part, that could send her into an insecure tailspin that will take that much longer to dig out of, so don't do it! My husband was the greatest! He said we could stay soft swap forever if that's what I wanted and it would be fine with him. It takes that kind of security for a woman to stick that foot out and gently test the waters. So, guys don't push!

If either spouse suddenly feels uncomfortable in any part of their new area of exploration, they need to immediately let their partner know so that they can talk about it. I remember the first time I saw my husband have intercourse with another woman. It seemed surreal. At the moment, it really didn't have much effect on me. It was a day or two afterwards that it started bugging me a bit and I needed that extra reassurance from him. I felt a comfort when he said we didn't have to have full swap with every couple we encountered and for us to be very selective in our approach to full swap. Aaaaaah..... That took the pressure off of me! I also realized when he came to me out of the blue and stated "You know, every time we get together with that couple, you don't have to fuck him." That statement also made me feel better

Communication is the key and taking it slow is important. Men need to be attentive to their wife's feelings and issues or you will never get anywhere in the Lifestyle. If her concerns are not addressed thoroughly by you both then they will eventually fester and cause problems at the most inappropriate times. I remember the first time I had an "issue" was when we were playing with two new couples a few months into the Lifestyle. The six of us had a lovely dinner at a Mexican restaurant and a few margaritas that loosened the verbal chatter. I noticed my husband concentrating his conversation with one of the two other wives. I could also tell she was also taken by my husband and witnessing this extended interest over conversation was a little unsettling emotionally, but logically I rationalized it away. This attentive attitude to other women was still fresh and new and I was still deciphering my feelings on all aspects. Since I am a bisexual female, I am used to showing and receiving interest from other females, too. This female was leaving me totally out of the conversation and targeting only my husband. A common guideline in the Lifestyle is for the two females to bond, so they feel comfortable sharing their husbands. This woman was not taking the steps to bond with me and concentrating 100% of her efforts on my husband and he was totally taking in the attention he was receiving. The other wife at the table was following correct etiquette and bonding with me and sharing conversation and stories to help us become comfortable with each other. Of course, by the time dinner was over, I was ready to allow this woman I had been talking with share my husband and I wasn't at all comfortable with the other woman who still was engaging my husband in conversation. Guess what happened once we all got back to the host's home. We were not in the house 60 seconds and my husband came from behind and slipped his hands under that woman's blouse that had monopolized him at the table. Needless to say, the next hour and a half she monopolizes his time to the point where the other wife got little time with him and I got a quick hug and hello when everyone finally decided to take a rest break. Normally, I would have been over there with my husband sharing his fun with him since I am bisexual, but every time I initiated sexual contact with her, she didn't say anything but also was non-responsive. I could tell she was really into my husband and couldn't get enough of him. My husband, playing with a female that was non-responsive to me, became a new uncomfortable issue for me. Was it right for me to be feeling this way? Logic said, "No." but I couldn't discount my emotions. That would be unhealthy. This was our first encounter with us playing with a straight woman. It was unsettling for me to not be welcomed and I had some feelings to address. Until I got my feelings sorted out on my reaction we had to stay away from straight women for some time.

Weeks after this play session we had several discussions and when the dust settled it was all due to with one fact only. She was not bisexual and the limitations that set in our play sessions made me feel cut off from my husband. Up until that point I had been able to be involved with every aspect of play with others so these were new feelings for me. Everyone has their issues and this one surfaced early for me. Like it or not, not all our issues are logical and it's irrelevant if they are not. Emotions aren't governed by logic – only your reactions to them. So, the important aspect is to recognize things that make you uncomfortable and discuss them with your partner before they morph into something bigger.

Chapter Three

MYTHS AND MISCONCEPTIONS

If you have problems in your marriage and you enter the Lifestyle, then the problems are usually going to be magnified.

It's no holds barred sex...

I believe one of the major things that has held back society at large over the years in acceptance of the Lifestyle, are the erroneous misconceptions about it. One of the largest misconceptions is that it is a no holds barred "free for all" for sex. People not in the Lifestyle many times think there are no limits and everyone plays with everyone else, with no rules or limitations. Both women and men outside the Lifestyle seem to harbor the thought that men control everything. When in reality, the entire Lifestyle is controlled by the women. I hate to say it guys, but many times you follow your wife around and she dictates. As I have mentioned before, one of the important aspects in the Lifestyle is for the women to bond. Think about it guys, what wife is going to allow another woman to play with her husband if she doesn't like the woman? If you keep playing with a woman that your wife dislikes, what kind of tension is that going to cause later at home when the two of you are alone? She will carry that thought and let it possibly fester inside. Let's face it ladies, logic doesn't always dictate in our world when the hormones are surging and the emotions can carry us off. A woman will start to feel that her husband doesn't respect her wishes and feel alienated from her husband when he is playing with the woman she doesn't like and it's most likely going to cause larger issues down the road for the two of you. I can't stress the fact that the two women must bond first and approve of each other before any activity commences. Guys, just keep it in perspective. Who is the most important one in your life? Obviously your wife is the most important person. At some point, before play can take place, the two females have to talk and decide if they like each other. It's not always a spoken thing either. Women use there instincts much more than men do. Many times I have approached a woman and just "felt" she wasn't for me. My husband, of course, is standing there dumbfounded thinking I'm crazy because he didn't see what was wrong with her. So men, if your wife decides she doesn't like the lady (even if she is a 10), cut your losses and move on. You don't want to tick your wife off and her slam the door shut to the whole evening. You can point out couples you are attracted to and then let your wife take it from there if she wants to pursue them. You both need to feel comfortable with others and unfortunately we women tend to be pickier than men.

Women are man handled...

A myth that many females have about the Lifestyle is that the men will carry them off into a corner and take advantage of them. Let's get something straight here ladies. The majority of clubs and parties only allow couples. Okay, now stop thinking with your emotions and think with your logic. What is going to happen when your husband grabs a woman out of nowhere and throws her over his shoulder and carries her off and takes advantage of her? You are going to slap him up side the head as soon as he throws the unwilling woman over his shoulder (okay maybe sooner than that). "Couples only" parties and clubs have the wives monitoring their own husband's behavior. Consequently, the men are all gentlemen. Now that's not to say that once in awhile you will sneak a jerk or two in there but they just aren't prevalent at all.

I remember one of the first times I encountered an ass at a party. It was a small house party and there were only about 6 couples in the apartment. I literally had not been in the apartment more than 3 minutes and as I was walking to the kitchen to say "Hello" to the hostess, this stranger walks up behind me (totally naked) and reaches around and grabs my hips and says, "Boy, do I have something for you." I turned around and hanging out of his mouth as he was talking to me was a condom packet. He grabbed the condom and shook it in front of my face. Now, there a lot of colorful responses I could have come back with but this was a very small party and it was going to be hard enough dodging this guy all night without making a total scene about the remark. I took the high road and said "No I'm not ready." I turned around and kept talking to the hostess. He immediately reached between my legs and rubbed my thigh and said, "You sure seem like you are ready to me." I then turned around and took a firmer approach, "No!" Finally, he got the message. Some guys get the hint fast and others you have to be direct and bang them over the head with it. Now, had this been a guy that I wanted to play with, I would have looked at his comment in a whole different light and I would have bantered with him (even though his approach was rude). Even though this was a small party and there was one asshole in the group, the evening turned out to be a great time. All the other couples were very fun and we both ended up playing with four of the six couples. It was at this party that I met a wife of one of the couples that became a regular playmate of ours. We played with both of them at the party, but as our friendship grew she was allowed to come and play at our house without her husband. She is one of the most assertive females I have ever run into and a delight to be around. Her husband travels a lot and was happy that she was in good hands when he was away.

A couple of months later, we ran into the same couple that had the asshole husband at another party (yes, it is a small world, even in Los Angeles). This time his wife had the "hots" for my husband and asked flat out for him to fuck her. Not really thinking of the consequences, my husband quickly agreed and bent her over the side the bed in the big group room we happened to be in with about 10 other people. He is just fucking away doggie style with her and guess who comes after me? Her husband, of course! I did some quick dancing around and then politely got distracted with someone else near me. Another lesson learned was our misconception that everyone played as individuals much like a single person. In the swinging world couples are many times seen as one unit, a team, so to speak. They aren't two individuals like singles, but come to play as a team. If you approach one of the team members, then both should be open to play or you just don't play unless you discuss it. Usually, the assumption is made that the approaching couple has already discussed and approved of both parties of the other couple before they approach them individually. My husbands' mistake in accepting her invitation was that he was opening up for me to play with her husband and I didn't want any part of her husband. There are always polite ways to get out of situations such as this, but the key is not to get in the middle of it in the first place. This requires some very open communication between partners when at a party.

Swing environments are seedy...

Another myth by many is that the home parties take place in low class seedy locations. I'm sure there are some of those out there but the majority of parties take place in middle class America homes or large estates. About half of the parties we attend here in Los Angeles, are at very nice multi-million dollar homes. They have great food and wine for everyone and some have a small cover charge at the door to cover the expenses. A friend of ours in Orange County has a swing group that gets together about once every 6 weeks. They have over three hundred couples as members of their group. You have to go through an interview process to join. You would never expect what goes on behind that suburbia front door. A very normal nice looking neighborhood with large yards and their three bedroom house has about 2000 square feet. When they have a party they send the kids to friends for the night and they do it up big. She cooks for about a week and has these lavish buffets with homemade lasagna, orange chicken, croissants, mini sandwiches, chocolate dipped strawberries and seafood dips etc. They have a full bar along with multi homemade spiked punches and as much variety as any commercial bar. They put up in their backyard a mosquito netting cabana with mattresses and pillows, tiki torches and soft lighting and even a blow up jumper room that's normally for kids. Having sex in a bouncing environment can't be passed up if you get the chance.

We rarely have seen parties within our own neighborhood until just recently. We saw a posting on one of the forum sites that there was a house party going on within two blocks of our home. There were over 500 people on the invite list and 150 had RSVP'd that they were attending. For the first time in three years we actually walked to a swing party.

Men ejaculate many times a night....

Let me startle you with an unexpected revelation I discovered quickly in the Lifestyle. The goal is usually not for men to orgasm until late in the evenings. We girls can cum over and over in an evening. Whereas, with the men, many times they don't ejaculate at all in the evening or at the very least they save it for the very end of the evening when ready to go home. Many men do not want any down time during the evening for fear they will miss out on playing with someone. If they ejaculate, then that guarantees there is going to be at least 20 minutes to over an hour of Mr. Empty Pants and his enthusiasm is definitely lowered. There are some men that are able to do repeat orgasms with short turn around times, but they are a minority at most parties. If you meet one – enjoy!

Ladies don't embarrass a man by insisting that you want him to cum if the evening is early. Most likely he will make excuses and get around it. Many men don't like to admit outright that they don't want to ejaculate because it will take them out of the game temporarily and they can't play right away. Now as the evening starts rolling up, then definitely tell them you want them to cum. By then, they will be more than happy to make your desires come true and at this point - orgasm will be the goal!

Only Women that are Sluts are in the Lifestyle...

I have met some of the most outwardly conservative women in the Lifestyle and you would never suspect they were Swingers. There are school teachers, school administrators, nurses, lawyers, doctors, counselors, realtors, bankers, loan officers, mortgage brokers, artists, security specialists, engineers, plumbers, children's autism specialist, film directors, actors, etc., in the Lifestyle. I think that every facet of society has a member present in the Lifestyle. They are all out there and represented. Don't feel shy. You are not the first of your field to be interested because someone else has beaten you to it. I have met some of the most educated and cultured ladies and men at parties. The women are Miss Etiquette on the outside and behind closed doors, a tigress on the inside. There have been a few "fridged" ones that disappointed us and carried their stiff upper lips into the play area, but for the most part these were far and few between.

Disease is prevalent...

The use of condoms is a must in the Lifestyle. Until the medical community comes up with a better alternative, the condom is the best protection against sexually transmitted diseases besides abstinence. Abstinence is the only 100% full proof method against disease. If you want to have a lot of sex you have to take on some degree of risk. Most swingers consider the risks extremely small.

Much smaller than out in the single dating world because the majority of swingers are life long couples that take care of themselves and hopefully are mature enough to not take unnecessary risks. There is a small percentage of members in the swinging community that go "bareback" or without a "raincoat" - sex without a condom. Many are men that have very large units and have a problem with condoms. There are small groups, also that over time have gotten to know the other couple and have played enough times with them that they feel they can trust them. In that case, always get an updated proof of no STD's and even that isn't definitive proof because it could take months after exposure for disease to develop.

The other question that comes to mind is very small majority of Lifestylers question that safety of oral sex and transmission of disease. I would suggest you ask your doctor if you are that concerned. From what research I have read on the subject, there is always is a small chance of transmission of disease from saliva through a sore on the penis or cut on the vagina but the actual documentation of this ever happening is so minute that my husband and I didn't consider it a factor that bothered us. You have to make a decision on on how much this issue really bothers you. We actually ran into a couple that was really to the point of having a psychosis on this subject and the last few times we played with them it really was just too much effort because we were required to put saran wrap over her to lick her pussy and to use a condom to give head to him. Once you go this far with it you look at one another and say "Gee, are these people really worth this?" My husband and I agreed that it was way too much effort and although we thought they were super people personally, they just didn't have it when it came to having sex with them because of their strong concerns.

You have to decide what risks you want to take. If you want zero percentage of risk then don't get in the Lifestyle. One thing that might reduce exposure even further is for a couple to stay only soft-swap and not have intercourse with other people. This definitely will help reduce the risks, but it doesn't eliminate them by any means. If you want to know exactly what the possible risks entail, I would recommend having an honest conversation with your Doctor.

Men have to fight off homosexual advances...

You know what? I think this fear is perpetuated by "homophobic men" in the Lifestyle. Then outsiders hear about it and get the wrong idea. For goodness sakes guys, get a grip on it! Just because another guy brushes up against your unit or balls during sex doesn't constitute he wants to have sex with you. Most likely you aren't his type. Okay, just kidding!

In the three years my husband and I have been playing I think we may have run across 6 couples that the male was open to more than just the usual female play. Sometimes you will get hints of it ahead of time in your E-mail conversations. Just because a guy likes his ass hole to be played with by his wife's fingers or special toys, does not mean he is bisexual. A lot of straight men like their asses played with because their semen manufacturing is in the prostate that is accessible through the ass or stimulation outside of the ass behind their scrotum. Stimulation of the prostate makes for major ejaculations and orgasm sensations. It's only natural for the male to enjoy added intensity to his orgasms.

Now there are a few guys out there (those 6 couples that we ran into during the 3 years) that want to perform oral or do full penetration. If this isn't your thing then just give them a polite, "No". Personally, one of my own fantasies is to see a guy give my husband a blow job. Even though my husband has no interest in this area, we still continue to talk about it because it always is a big turn on for me.

It really is a double standard in the Lifestyle that female bisexually is so accepted but men being bi isn't as widely accepted. Not many men put it out there on the front page of their profile and the ones that I have run into that state they are bisexual are many times only into the oral. Maybe sometime in the future people won't be so judgmental and this old double standard will slowly fade away. I don't think it's any person's business on what others choose as a sexual orientation. I believe people need to only govern themselves because they don't have the qualifications to govern others, since they haven't lived their lives.

Only couples with marital problems are in the Lifestyle...

There seems to be only a small percentage of couples we have encountered that are in the Lifestyle for all the wrong reasons. If you have problems in your marriage and you enter the Lifestyle, then the problems are usually going to get more magnified. The issues in the Lifestyle will draw out your weak points and you will eventually have to address those issues. I am happy to say that the huge majority of couples we meet are in the Lifestyle for the right reasons. They are not there to fix their marriages, but only to enhance an already great marriage and add some zing. The Lifestyle experiences have a tendency to draw you closer together, when your marriage is good and on a solid foundation, Couples share intimate experiences both good and bad and you talk about them and explore options together. This kind of intimate talk draws people closer and they start exposing their inner likes and dislikes. You get to see what makes your mate tick and what really also upsets them. Many times they aren't overt about it and it's just the generally later comments after the fact, that are brought up and you realize that had they not brought it up it wouldn't have been weighing heavy on their mind. I remember one time I participated in a sex game at one of the parties we attended. I volunteered for both games being one as a contestant and the other as a judge. I think this surprised my husband because he brought it up twice in the next 24 hours. It meant nothing in my mind except to have fun at a party with no arterial motive involved. When my husband brought it up a couple times later, it made me think he had some questions about it. Talk about things and get through any issues that may be on the others' mind. As we know, we can all twist things around to make something out of nothing. Many times emotion has no logic. Take your partner's concerns seriously no matter how small they might seem. If you ignore little concerns they will become big concerns later.

Bi women can't control themselves around straight women...

This one really flabbergasts me every time I run into it. I will talk more about the differences between the two in a later chapter but this misconception is one that definitely has to be addressed. We have encountered many straight women that think that if they play with a couple whose female is bisexual, that the bi girl won't be able to resist the straight girl. Ladies, I am here to tell you straight from a bisexual female's mouth, that it couldn't be farther from the truth. Who wants to give attention to another person that doesn't want the attention? I don't want to try and pleasure a woman that has no interest in me. What is the point of that? That would be like a straight woman wanting to pleasure a man that doesn't want to have anything to do with her. That is no fun! Please understand that the cock is many times number one in a bisexual females' life! She is going after the cock just like you are but the icing on her cake is to play with the female, but the female is by no means the cake!

Now, for those rare bisexual females that decide they are going to try and turn a straight woman, I have a few words for you. You are rude and it's totally unacceptable for you to approach a straight woman with those intentions. You give us good bi girls a bad name and I'm damn tired of it!

You have to have intercourse with other couples to be in the Lifestyle...

Not true. Soft swapping is totally accepted in the Lifestyle and many couples never venture any further than soft swap for various reasons. So to experience the erotic environment of swinging does not mean you have to actually have intercourse with other people.

Chapter Four

CONVINCING
THE WIFE

The security of your love, affection and devotion will allow her to open her boundaries up and start experimenting further with bigger aspects of the Lifestyle.

I have had many men approach me and ask the number one question, "How do I get my wife interested in the Lifestyle?" "How do I approach her without her freaking out on me?" Okay men, listen up, because I'm going to give you the secrets in this chapter to follow and entice your wife or love partner into the Lifestyle (this also works for women wanting to approach their husbands). If your wife is like most you will need to easy into it and not just say, "Hey, have you ever thought of us having sex with another couple?" There are very few women that I would recommend this direct of an approach.

One of the first things to do is to start openly talking about *her* fantasies (your fantasies will come later). One of the important aspects of the approach is not for her to feel threatened. You don't want her thinking that she isn't enough for you and you need added stimulation in your life because she just doesn't do it for you anymore. She may jump to this conclusion if you immediately start talking about what *you* want. Everything needs to revolve around her and you making her happy by new experimentation and experiences. Most women will have a tough time at first verbalizing their desires because honestly many of them have never taken the time to actually analyze them. If she has problems coming up with anything then you need to start prompting her by asking her questions. Here are ideas that should help get the ball rolling and you can expound on top of her answers with what limited information she is going to give you in the beginning.

Tell her that you would love it if she didn't wear panties sometime when you are going out for dinner and she allows you feel her pussy in public under the table. Ask her if this sounds exciting. If she says, "Yes", then expand on it with more questions on the how, when and where potentials of the situation. If she answers, "No", then ask her what part of the situation makes her uncomfortable. Is it the possible exposure? Nine out of ten times this is the culprit and a woman has to feel secure that there is no chance of anyone seeing it happening. Otherwise, she is a "slut" in her mind (but we know different). Once she gets comfortable with the ideas of these types of limited situations, she will then advance to wanting to do it in a more open environment with the possibility of exposure. The thrills have to start out small and slowly advance as she becomes accustom to the little things and want bigger things. Make plans to go out and actually do this fantasy and get your wife open to fulfilling different fantasies. You have to start in small steps and then advance forward. If she immediately starts asking you what your fantasies are then get around the question. Don't tell her *your* fantasies yet! Tell her that you get excited by seeing her get excited. Your fantasy is to help her live out her fantasies and you explore together new experiences together. This will be very true for you and it's a non-threatening answer to her. Your foundation needs to be set for her and not for you. If she pulls a fast one on you and won't allow you to do these in a public place then start by doing things in your own private back yard. Experiment in doing her in the garage behind the car, but leave the door open, so no one walking by can see you. Another good one is to reach over in the car and fondle her while stuck in traffic.

Spend a couple weeks on playing out some of these small fantasies for her and then advance to doing them in more public areas. Once she is comfortable with the little stuff she will seek bigger thrills. Take her in the department store and go in to the dressing room and play together. Remember to make it all about her. The ultimate goal is for her to feel secure with you in a public place and your genuine desire of seeing her get excited.

As your little escapades get more daring for the two of you in public then it will become time to bring up your fantasies. It's important to do these things in public or semi public areas so she gets used to other people being around, since the Lifestyle is based on others being around. The part of the Lifestyle that should be brought up at this point is watching and being watched. Don't ask her for more interest in anything except these two things. Ask her if it would be exciting for the two of you to be playing with one another in the dark corner of a bar when another couple next to you realizes what you are doing and they are watching you. Tell her that the woman's' husband has reached up his own wifes' dress and is fondling her while watching the two of you. Tell her that they can't see her kitty because the skirt is covering everything, but they can see that you have your hand between her legs. Tell her she is getting very wet and excited and you would love to turn her around and pull her dress up from behind and enter her while standing there without making any movements, so no one will know that you are inside her. Then concentrate on what the other couple is doing. Go into detail on what he is doing to his wife in front of you and what she is doing and how they are reacting. These mental exercises will help her get used to the idea of other people being around and exposed to watching and being watched.

After you have had a few of these real life fantasies lived out you should interject the possibility of the other woman touching her. Tell her that the husband told you in the bathroom earlier that his wife is bisexual and finds your wife very attractive and she would just like to feel her breasts and your wife doesn't have to reciprocate in any manner. Just start dropping suggestions in this area to see if she shows any interest in another woman touching her. Then tell her that her husband would like to reach over and feel her breasts and see how she responses to that. Keep the activity on your wife and her wants and desires. By his time, she will be open enough with you that if she wants to expand things and ask you if you would like certain things to happen then be honest with her but don't make them any big deal and always steer the conversation back towards her and you wanting to see her excited and stimulated.

Keep the focus off yourself. This constant reinforcement of the activities centering on your wife and not you gives your wife the security she needs regarding your affections. Women can become threatened very easily by their husbands' fantasies and desires and if they think these activities are going to center around him then the whole deal is going to slip down the drain rapidly. Every woman knows that men are horny and usually want to experiment with other women, but for a woman to allow her husband to do that she must feel 100% satisfied that she is top queen bee and no one comes close to fulfilling his desires. Make sure she knows you think exactly that and remind yourself that she is number one and her happiness is the only thing that is important. The security of your love, affection and devotion will allow her to open her boundaries up and start experimenting further with bigger aspects of the Lifestyle.

It will be at this time that you might want to suggest setting up a website and meeting other couples and go to a swing club nearby if one is available. Never keep her in the dark and when you have potential couples to meet. You need to first run them by her to see if she thinks they would be acceptable. Mental head games can rapidly get out of control if you are keeping things from her and she finds out things through Emails and IM's by surprise. No one wants surprises and unexpected things seem to make people think that they weren't told these things for a reason. That reason is never a positive one, no matter how you try to explain it. You will also need to set up personal boundaries prior to meeting anyone - what you will and will not do. There may be a few issues with you, but for the most part these boundaries are going to come from her. You will need to talk about potential jealousy issues that may arise. This is very important to stay in close communication and reinforce your love for your wife. Jealousy gets out of control when the woman feels her husband has forgotten about her because his concentration is so focused on the other woman. Another big culprit for jealousy to pop up is not enough free time at home to concentrate just on each other. You can't go out playing with others when your sex at home is neglected in any way. Your mate always comes first in order for the Lifestyle to work for you as a couple.

Chapter Five

WOMEN'S CONCERNS

It is always customary for a man outside the playgroup to ask first if he can touch a female.

Where do I start? We women have so many issues and it really compounds our worries in the Lifestyle. Hopefully, I can put many of your concerns at ease. Let's face it, if we aren't at ease with the whole concept and situation then our guys with the raging hard-ons can just forget it! No amount of talk is going to convince us to participate, if we don't have a few questions answered!

Younger women mean younger bodies...

One of the biggest hesitations a woman has is displaying her body with all its faults out there for others to see. Very few women are blessed with perfect bodies. If you are a woman with a perfect body, "Bite me!" Most women have extra padding here and there and work hard at keeping most of the extra padding off. As we age, it takes more effort to achieve the same effect. Damn, I remember the days in my twenties that I could eat everything I wanted and not do any exercise and still be a size 5. Those were the good old days! Now I have to exercise, however, and watch my diet and lose about half a pound a week-if I'm lucky. Plus, if I want sculptured muscles then I have to lift weights. It use to be fashionable and acceptable for a woman not to have any muscle definition and then some bitch years back spoiled it for all of us. Now it's less acceptable and we have to workout like maniacs. Gee, now that I think about it we were even able to be a size 14 and that was sexy and acceptable. Don't forget that Marilyn Monroe wasn't a size 5! Ladies, all sizes and shapes are acceptable in the Lifestyle and you will have no problem in finding playmates. It's all attitude. I am a curvy woman and as much as I try, my genetics lean towards the size 10 category. I have found men really love curves and they find them sexy as hell. A full round ass and curvy breasts can make men drool. You don't have to be a string bean to get plenty of attention. Also if you are packing a lot more extra pounds don't despair because I have seen women over the 200lb category have the men lined up. There is something for everyone. I personally prefer women in the 135lb and up category. Below that weight, I feel like I'm hugging a bag of bones. I don't really care for that if I have a choice. Everyone has their favorites, so ladies, just because you don't have a perfect body don't discount yourself. If you line up (what you think) ten perfect looking women, you'll get complaints from everyone of them down the line about their own bodies. We all do it and the funny thing is that the majority of men still get a hard on for us. It's the "strange" pussy that can be a huge turn on for them, regardless of the details of the container. So look in the mirror and say, "I'm one sexy lady!" Then go out and play with that attitude. It's all in the attitude anyway.

Wardrobe...

Every woman knows that if you don't feel good in what you are wearing then you are going to be preoccupied with the way you look instead of concentrating on the moment. First off you need to go out and buy you a few new items to play in that you are happy with and fit perfectly. Every party dictates it's own theme or clothing parameters. You really have three types of clothing for Lifestyle parties. You have street clothes, lingerie and costumes. All of them need to exude eroticism. Show your assets and highlight them. If you have great legs wear really short outfits and if it's great breasts then show tons of cleavage! Generally for home parties, I dress a bit more conservative if I don't know the hosts. I will wear a micro short skirt that is easy to get in an out of and a form fitted, off the shoulder top, that is very tight and that outlines my breasts. I don't wear panties or a bra. Yes, I do realize that these are two very sexy pieces of lingerie, but they also hinder playful activities. There is nothing more aggravating than caressing a woman and having a little foreplay and reaching to feel her breasts and they are so tightly wrapped up you can't get your fingers in there! I have even seen women wear merry widows and you can't get access at all to the nipples. I don't wear panties because I can never find them when I am getting dressed after playing in low lighting. I don't know how many times I have had my husband standing there waiting on me and I'm still getting dressed because I have to hunt down all the pieces and parts of my clothing. The clothing is never where you put it. In the middle of all the activities in the room someone else has laid their stuff on top of yours or moved it because they were doing the bump and grind right there. As far as I'm concerned, the less pieces and parts the better.

For parties where you know the hosts or for commercial swing clubs, you can dress in lingerie or more revealing outfits. I enjoy the see through lace tube dresses that you can just slip off and on easily. Most high end lingerie stores carry these types of outfits or you can order them on line. I recently bought a black dress that was made of the stretch material and it had a plunging neck line almost down to my navel. Outfits such as this are easily ordered over the internet and many outfits are under forty dollars.

Many of the parties you attend will have themes. This, of course, gives each woman the excuse to go buy a costume to fit the theme. There are websites that just have sexy costumes. I recently attended a Dirty Doctor and Naughty Nurses party and I think I found about 30 different nurses outfits on one website. All were revealing and sexy and it was a tough decision on which one to go with when the time came to place the order. I finally decided on a black vinyl outfit and was the evil nurse of the group. Above all please wear shoes you can walk in and that don't take 15 minutes to take off or put back on. Your husband might appreciate it. My husband just hates having to hang around watch me fumble with the straps on my shoes. The lighting is always low and it's very difficult to see the holes in the dark. Plus, after you have had a cocktail or two it becomes increasingly difficult to walk in those 5 inch spiked heels. The spiked heels look sexy but they become a hindrance and mine ended up collecting dust in the closet. Wear the thicker heels, ladies, and go for safety and comfort, if possible.

Hygiene ...

Don't laugh, but there are actually people who go out to play and don't shower first. Personally, I have been lucky enough not to encounter them, but have seen complaints on other people's website profiles referencing this exact topic. People please show some class and clean up before you go play. No one wants body odor or sweaty smells hitting them in the face. That's a real turn off and you are going to get turned down without question. Just what every woman wants to encounter – a guy that smells like the back end of a horse.

Ladies you have a lot to do to get ready to play. So, let's just go through the list. Get your nails done and don't forget a pedicure. A lot of people are going to be inches from your toes so don't forget to make them pretty. Also, make sure you put a new blade in your razor, because you don't want to make any mistakes down there. Get some shaving cream instead of just soap, so it will soften your skin and make it easier to shave the hair. Now before you jump in the shower you need to tweeze those brows (if you didn't have them done) and pull out any stray nipple hairs (Eeeek....you know the ones).   Once finished, jump in the shower and get started washing and conditioning your hair then start on the hard stuff. For those of you women who don't have thick course hair and can go to the salon and have a bikini wax done - then please do it. Otherwise, join us poor souls that have so much hair that every time I had a waxing done I could still see enough hairs to braid a twelve foot strand. Waxing never gets 100% of the hairs and if you want baby smooth absolutely hair free you have to shave (forget the fact you have to let the hair grow out before it's waxed again). Yuk! So, shave your bikini area all the way up to the navel if necessary. Leave a nice strip of hair down there so it's nicely manicured or just shave it all off. Make sure and lift each leg up high so you can shave the lips and the inside of the lips. Yes, there are a lot of hairs on the inside of those lips for many ladies, so be careful! Now, its time to give some attention to your back side and make sure all the fur is gone. No one wants to see a hairy ass. I guarantee you there is hair around your ass button and if you don't believe me go get a mirror! Shave the inside of your cheeks and all around your button and both butt cheeks if it's warranted. You natural blondes have it so good! Even blondes, however, may have a lot of hair but it's not as apparent because of the color. So, get rid of it if you have too much. Clean and trimmed up is the goal. I shave my enter unit every morning in the shower. It's the same as shaving my legs or my underarms. Just something you do every day so there is no stubble. Most ladies have problems in the beginning with razor bumps. Just go to a beauty supply store and pick up an expensive blue bottle of liquid stuff made just for razor bumps. It works wonders! A fresh shave is absolutely mandatory because no one wants facial burns going down on you with stubble. Once I went down on a woman and I know it had been at least 24 hours since she shaved so I didn't spend near the time down in the southern hemisphere as I had wanted but I couldn't take the friction on my lips and mouth anymore. She was going to rub my mouth raw with those bristles. Please ladies have a little more consideration. Licking sandpaper is not my idea of a good time. Neither is coming up with a mouth full of hair. For those women that think we are still in the '70's – we aren't! Retro bushes are not in fashion. You need to bring that bush up to date with all the edges neatly trimmed and if you leave any hair at all down there then make sure you comb it out first so you get all the stragglers. No one likes hair in their food. That really has a tendency to destroy the mood just a tad.

Make sure you floss along with using your toothpaste. You would be surprised at the amount of people that forget their breath mints. Last but not least, please exfoliate, exfoliate, and exfoliate! Get a long handle brush and soap it up and scrub your back (and your legs, arms, stomach, butt). Nothing is worse than caressing a person's skin and feeling those little invisible bumps on the skin. It makes you want to scratch them off them. Yuck! So, don't forget to use the brush everywhere or buy some of those special creams that have built in granules to buff you smooth. Once out of the shower lather on the moisturizer and make your skin feel like velvet.

Etiquette...

There is a certain amount of unique etiquette involved in swinging One of the major etiquette rules that we have already touched on but will go into more detail is the acceptance of playing with one half of the team and the other half assumes they will be included. It's a natural assumption and one you should not forget. If you approach a woman and want to play with her then her male partner will assume he can play with you. So, if you don't want to have this assumption going on then you must spell it out that you are interested in her but your wife is not interested in playing with her husband. Most likely nine out of ten times, the couple will decline your offer. Everyone that plays as a team will want to do exactly that – play as a team. Singling out one of the team members is not acceptable to most couples. That is why it is so important for both of you to agree on both of the partners on a team. This brings up a fact that many of you will eventually find out on your own. There are a lot of beautiful older women out there that have kept up their looks, go to the spa and obviously spend a lot of money on their appearance, whereas their male partner looks his age. He has a stomach and is bald and hasn't kept his muscle tone. This is where communication between the two of you is vital and you must agree on couples as a whole. It doesn't matter guys if the other wife is drop dead gorgeous if her male partner is substandard in your terms. Your wife won't approve of the situation and neither should you think about asking her. Just think about if the reverse were true.

What if the male partner was Mr. Atlantis with muscles and pecks and his wife has 3 chins and a donut roll around her waist? Come on now, there are no decisions to be made and obviously you need to remember both aspects of the equation equal a whole. You do need to stay aware of the fact that first impressions don't always prove to be true later. Many times we have met couples where I initially was not attracted but once I spent a few minutes talking to them my attitude started changing because they really had playful fun attitudes. Don't ever discount personality because we know it can really be hot!

Another problem that is chronic in the Lifestyle is a lack of understanding that you hold appointments and meetings with people the same as outside the Lifestyle. If you cannot meet at the required time, then you simply call ahead of time and give your apologizes. You would not believe the number of people that flake and just never show up at a party or dinner and don't call and let the hosts know about their problem. This issue seems to be a high problematic area in the Lifestyle and you need to give your prospective "dates" a heads up when you have an emergency arise. This is only a courtesy and you obviously would want the same done to you if one of your dates flaked on meeting.

I'm frozen in the carpool lane...

It always amazed my husband when we attended parties, that I would get this glazed look over my eyes and not be able to focus on everything. He coined the phrase, "I was stuck in the carpool lane". My brain was moving 200mph and I was overwhelmed with stimulus. A beautiful woman would walk by us and give me the look (whatever look I don't know) and my husband would ask if I saw her. I would respond with "Huh?" He would say, "That woman is interested in you - go and talk to her." I of course would say, "What the heck are you talking about?" I swear every time he would be right. I was clueless and pretty much still am today. I completely rely on my husband to field interest for me. Maybe it's all those thousands of years of males pursuing women that they recognize the slightest cues. Whatever it is, I know I don't have it. He will say, "Did you see how she/he kept looking over here?" Of course my response is always, "No, I didn't notice it." I think his radar is on high alert and recognizes these key components in the sexual dance because many times I just don't see it, even when it's pointed out I don't see it. Consequently, I always trust my husband's radar and not my own because his is super charged with atomic power and mine just runs on the old AA batteries.

How do I avoid those I don't want to play with...

Now for men, this is usually not a problem but women have a tendency to be more polite when avoiding the undesirables. On email we all know this is not a problem. You just reply that you don't think you are a good match and give them good luck wishes and send them on their merry way. It's the avoidance, however, at parties that can be the real stickler of getting out of situations gracefully. Many of you will just take the direct approach and won't care how insulting you may sound to the other person and just be blatant about your disapproval of them. I like to take the more classy approach with other people, because I prefer people to respond to me the way I would respond to them. There is a fine line of being direct and just plain rude. So, if you think you can be direct without being rude, then go for it.

For those of you that feel uncomfortable with directness there are a few ways that are subtle, but still get the meaning across and won't come off being rude. Make polite conversation and when the question comes up asking you to play just say maybe later because you are just wanting to rest right now (provided you had been playing previously in the evening). One of the most uncomfortable situations can be when you are in the middle of playing with two or three couples and one of the partners you aren't interested in starts caressing you and showing interest. One of easiest ways out is to pull away like you didn't notice and immediately start playing with your own partner. Taking shelter with your partner usually halts advancements of others. If that doesn't do it then just look at them and gives a polite "No, Thank you." Many women have a hard time saying "No" to someone and being that assertive. A lot of times it's this one aspect of having to say "No" that women fear in group play and that's why they don't go to parties. They don't want to be put in the situation of having to be assertive about the situation.

One other alternative is to use code words with your mate and when they recognize that you are uncomfortable then they can take action for you. The best thing, however, is always just being assertive on your own and stand up for yourself. As hard as that may be for you, you definitely need to acquire a thick skin when playing with strangers or new acquaintances. Rarely have I ever seen anyone object to a simple, "No".

Helen Keller Sex...

It is always customary for a man outside the playgroup to ask first if he can touch a female. There are times, however, when you aren't playing just one on one with another couple, but due to the location (on a king size bed) where there are several couples on the bed - then it's pretty much a lot of open groping. My husband calls it "Helen Keller Sex". If you get in a situation that you don't want someone to touch you then just politely say "No" to them. One thing I've found in the Lifestyle is that people are very respectful of others and they know that "No" means "No" with no questions asked.

This Helen Keller sex is the main reason many people shy away from group play. I have found that a large percentage of people prefer to play just one on one privately. It allows them to concentrate solely on the individual (couple) and not be interrupted by outsiders. They are able to control and dictate easier and not have any unwanted advances in their play. There are even couples that take this play to the most extreme and they play in separate rooms from their mate. There seems to be a definite preference by couples. They either like to play in the same room as their mate or separate rooms. Personally, my husband and I enjoy the visual stimulus of others playing. There are couples, however, that prefer isolation because of the Helen Keller sex factor and they don't like the distractions that a group situation will bring. There certainly is no right or wrong way of playing but as you progress in your swinging you will find that you have an affinity towards one or the other. Many couples that play in separate rooms do so because they find hearing their mate very distracting and don't feel like they can really open up and be freely themselves. I don't understand this concept, because I would think that no matter who you are playing with (spouse or otherwise) that you would be yourself. So, your playing methods shouldn't change just because your spouse is absent in the room. It does take different methods for different people, however, and if this works for you then certainly cultivate it. The unique aspect of the Lifestyle is that you have fun and respect others. There are no right and wrong ways in your playing. Just understand that certain rules and guidelines you may prefer may hinder you finding others that are also suitable for play.

When playing in group situations (more than with one other couple), the dynamics can change in the playing. Also the rules may change just a tad, but not by much because of the nature of the situation. When there are "puppy piles" of people in one bed, a person needs to be a bit more open to the possibility of others interacting with them while they are playing with the main person in front of them (or behind them). Men are supposed to always ask if they can touch you but many times just body language is used and words are not needed. Reading body language can be difficult and there are some people like myself, who never seem to pick up on the subtle hints people give off. When a group of naked people are all intermingling in a pile of bodies it's not uncommon for a female to reach over and caress someone and look to see their reaction. Sorry guys, but it's a double standard for males and it's always recommended that you ask permission to touch. If the person smiles at your caress and doesn't say anything then you would take that as a positive and continue while they are still in the middle of playing with someone else. For example, a woman may be mounted from behind by a male and another male will come up and stand in front of her. If she gives a positive reaction then he is open to pursue thing further. He may then move toward her head to see if she will grab his cock and then start giving him oral.

It takes a certain amount of aggression in a female to verbalize what she wants and needs. Sometimes the only time it's really easy for females to verbalize is when she firmly means "No". Many women would freak out if a man that they don't find attractive is touching them in any manner. If you have this problem then group play may not be as much fun. Your radar is always going to have to be on and it will be exhausting. I'm one of those women that can handle any man touching my arms, shoulders, back and breasts. It doesn't matter what he looks like and I will usually allow a man to touch and fondle my breasts. If I don't find him attractive, however, then that's all he will get to do and I won't allow him to proceed any further. This happens to be my own boundaries and I have found that not many woman hold to this openness. The majority of woman I have found won't allow a man to touch her anywhere if she has no intentions of playing with him. I happen to find some level of attraction to most men and women at least enough to tease and be playful, but may not find enough attraction to actually allow him (her) to do a full swap.

What do I do with the other woman...

When women first get in the Lifestyle and think about playing and the different scenarios they start to wonder what are they supposed to do with the other woman when they are playing in a group or just with one other couple. Well, obviously that depends if you have any interest in women in a sexual sense. There are no cut and dry levels of being bi and everyone has their own definition and boundaries. If you are a straight woman and have no interest in any sexual interaction with the other female then you will need to be up front about that prior to playing and you will concentrate all your efforts on the other man. Do not assume that when you tell a person that you are straight that they will think you don't want any sexual play with the female. I have known many women that classify themselves as straight and will allow a female to go down orally on them or they will kiss and fondle their breasts. Like I said before, there are all different interpretations of what the different labels are on people.

How do I initiate and be assertive...

This is a problem with a lot of females. We are used to being pursed and not having to be assertive. The Lifestyle warrants the female to be assertive since it's virtually run by the women. Being assertive can be a completely foreign thing to a woman. I had never been assertive in the past, until I ventured into the Lifestyle. Then I quickly saw that if we were going to play any given evening at a club that I was going to have to walk up and initiate. That was terrifying and still doesn't come naturally to me. I still have to push myself in every situation. It is something I constantly have to battle with and stay cognizant of in the Lifestyle. I know my husband will be perceived as "pushy" by women (which is many times a major turn off of theirs) if he goes up to a woman and initiates the conversation and playful talk. Clubs are a difficult place to go to if you are both shy. That's really why many people don't like clubs and prefer the one on one method of meeting through the emails and phone calls. This safe route is used because they know the couple in question is already interested in them at the point of setting up a meeting. There is no guessing involved, whereas, at a club environment this is always in question until you strike up a conversation and see where it leads. This is the aspect that holds many people back from that club environment. If you can overcome this possible hurdle, then the club can reap many rewards. More often than not, meeting one on one with a couple can be very frustrating. There are the no shows, the flakes, the liars and the fact that "all eyes are on you" syndrome. Being in this spotlight can be very intimidating. This is one reason that my husband and I don't like meeting and playing one on one with just a couple because I can't stand all eyes on me. There is nowhere to hide. In a crowd I can disappear if I choose, but in a one on one there is no where to go.

I could be replaced...

A fear of many women is the thought that once playing with others, their mate could replace them. Don't kid yourself ladies this fear also runs through your partners mind too. One of the most important aspects of playing is to be doing it for the correct reasons. The wrong reason would be to fix a problematic marriage. You must have a deeply loving relationship already prior to going into the Lifestyle. The Lifestyle should be used as just icing on the cake for your relationship. You need a solid foundation for your relationship which will only increase in love as experiences increase in the Lifestyle. One of the unique things that you already know, but will become very apparent, is that your loving spouse cannot be matched by any other person. They know you better than any other person and they love you. That deep emotional connection is what sets you apart from all the others you play with in the Lifestyle. Make no mistake and understand this important aspect that there will always be prettier, more handsome, better bodies, and better techniques by someone else. You are not the "be all" and "end all" in techniques in the Lifestyle and neither is your body. There is always someone better. That person is just a shell, however, compared to your spouse and they are the person that you have the deep emotional ties and devotion to and the "Mr/Mrs Perfect" is just a façade to you. This is important to remember in that you are not going to be replaced, unless you have a marriage that is already crippled. You only go into the Lifestyle to enhance an already close loving relationship.

Reading body language...

You would think with everyone on the same page in wanting to have sex that there wouldn't be so many subtle messages used. The majority, however, is only comfortable with passive suggestions and won't go out on a limb and be obvious about anything. We are all looking for playmates and although you run the risk of being rejected, it does make things so much easier when you are open and honest with other people. People really do need to develop a thicker skin in the Lifestyle and understand that when people reject you that they are rejecting a façade of you – not the "real" you.   Don't take things so personal.   You can't possibly please everyone, so don't expect everyone to like you.   One person may only like women that part their hair on the left side, so don't take offense if you aren't their cup of tea for the evening.   There are too many people that will be happy to play with you, so accept their decision with grace and move on.   There is something for everyone here in the Lifestyle and whatever you may be looking for I'm sure you will be able to find it.

When playing within a group, there are subtle clues that you need to be aware of.   Body positioning is a big factor.   If I see a man crawling towards me and I'm not interested I will turn my back to him or my husband may put himself in between us and there becomes a visual barrier. Someone turning their back to you can be a big sign that they don't want to play. Then if all else fails you will hear a "No thank you" from them.   Many men think if a woman leaves her ass sticking up in the air, she is interested in someone playing with her. Unfortunately, some men make assumptions and that gets them in trouble. Never assume when it comes to touching a woman. I have learned that it's best to keep my ass down or up against the wall so no one can come up behind me unexpectedly.   If you stick that ass up you will be constantly bombarded with hopeful playmates wanting to accommodate you so be forewarned with that body signal.

How do I deal with Thumpers...

I call men that act like they will never play again with another female in their entire life, a Thumper. I'm sure you know the type. Remember the little rabbit in one of the children's movies that has the foot that thumps with nervous energy. They can't wait to get their hands on you and are afraid you are going to be taken away from them so they have to get all they can get in a short amount of time. Guys, if you want women to be attracted to you then don't appear to be desperate no matter how desperate you really may be. They will almost be stalking you and you will get that sleazy feeling from them. Stay cool guys and simmer down or you are going to get turned down. If a guy starts irritating you and isn't cool, just excuse yourself from the conversation and go find your husband. Too often I think that the Thumpers were the boys that got picked last when playing in recess as a kid. I find Thumpers very irritating, but the one person that finds them more irritating than me is my husband. He can see a Thumper coming from 12 blocks away and has him pegged way before he gets in my line of sight. The Thumper really exhausts my husband's natural good nature.

Small clit syndrome...

Are you worried you won't be able to have an orgasm? There are a lot of distractions going on around you in the beginning when you first start playing. There are many women that cannot orgasm at all with anyone but their spouse. Over the course of many females I have found that in many cases (but not all...nothing's 100%) females that have an unusually large clit never seem to have a hard time reaching orgasm. So, my husband coined the phrase of "small clit syndrome" for women that under no circumstances appear to be getting close to orgasm. You can turn them upside down and whistle show tunes and they don't even moan. These "fridged" females seem to be there for their husbands and not for themselves. Don't ever swing just because it's your husband's idea. That's not fair to yourself or anyone around you. To make matters worse, most people can see right through you and won't want to play, unless you show genuine interest and enthusiasm. Both parties should be embracing the idea of swinging or you don't swing. If a woman cannot relax when playing with another person then it's only going to lead to frustration on everyone's part. Eventually, you may also grow some animosity against your spouse for the swinging, but in reality no one is to blame but yourself. If you swing then you choose to swing and no one else is to blame. So, if you start having uncomfortable feelings about swinging, immediately set your mate down and have a heart to heart discussion about your concerns. Only communication will resolve your problems and there is no such thing as too much communication. Swinging can bring a close relationship even closer but it will wedge a vast crevice in between two people if they aren't on the same page about their playing.

Jealousy issues...

I put this topic under the women's concerns but this is also a man's concern too. One of the largest issues and drama that arises in the Lifestyle are jealousy issues. If you can't deal with your jealousy issues then you have absolutely no business being in the Lifestyle. Now, granted many times you truly don't know how you are going to react in new situations until you have tried them. If the green eyed monster pops its head up then quietly deal with it and make no drama. Later talk to your spouse about how you felt and try and figure out the core reason that jealousy entered into the situation.

The husband of a new couple in the Lifestyle recently told me that he had a problem with his wife. If he stated to her, that he had no interest or affection towards a prospective female, his wife would practically force the other woman on him if she wanted to play her husband. When the same husband truly had interest and affection towards the other female, however, his wife would have a fit and refuse to play with the couple and want to go home. It was obvious that she was dealing with some insecurity issues and the two of them needed to talk things out. She wasn't being fair to her spouse insisting he play with someone he didn't want to play with and her jealousy was obvious when he met a woman that he truly had interest in. It seemed to them the only play situation that never had any drama to it was the MFM threesome. She liked being the center of attention. So happens the husband happened to be bi-curious, so he also got his attention and this became their solution to her jealousy issues. She simply couldn't deal with genuine likeable partners for her husband so they had to set their boundaries to just threesomes.

DOIN ONE FOR THE TEAM

Chapter Six

MEN'S CONCERNS

If you have a hard time dealing with rejection then you are going to have a hard time in the Lifestyle.

Men definitely don't have the concerns that women seem to have in the Lifestyle. They are rarely worried about wardrobe or hygiene and usually are only worried about the basics. There are few things, however, that have popped up with my dealing with men and they are indeed very specific to men. My husband has the attitude of, "Oh just get your clothes off!" I think many men share this direct to the point attitude, but if you do a little digging you will uncover a few things that do "bug" them from time to time.

How did my 9 inch cock shrink to 5 inches...

The number one concern men have is the size of their package. How does it measure up to everyone else out there? One of the most important things you can do is be honest about your unit size. If it's really 5 inches then don't say its 7 inches. Believe me, the other woman will be able to tell the difference and she may embarrass you by telling you that someone stole your 2 inches. Does size matter? Yes, to some degree. Most women consider anything from 5 to 7 inches normal. If you are above that or below it then you need to be honest. Every woman has a different definition of what is hung. I happen to think anything 8 inches and above as to being large. Some women think anything over 9 inches. We all have our own definition. Some prefer girth to length and you can't anticipate what a woman prefers unless you ask her. They like different things for different reasons. Some ladies have a very short canal and want a smaller cock when others can take a steamship. I'm not going to kid you and give the cliché of knowing how to use it being the most important aspect. You are going to find some women that definitely prefer a certain size and won't consider outside that framework. If you don't fall into her specifications then move on and don't sweat it. There will be plenty of women that do fall into your specs. One of the problems with size is the fact there are a lot of guys out there that have large cocks and they do know how to use them, so to state the old cliché really doesn't cut it.

Recently, I heard of a female player that was told by the male of the other couple that he had an 8 inch unit. This new couple decided to play in separate rooms and consequently the inexperienced new female swinger was left alone with the male and to her surprise he undressed and exposed a full erection of 4 inches. She proceeded to play with him for 4 hours. Whew! She felt obligated and that really compounded the problem. She was afraid to go to interrupt her husband and let him know that she had been lied to and that she didn't want to play with the guy. Obviously, as a new couple in swinging, you can't second guess every scenario that you will run in to, but you should never be afraid of interrupting your spouse to let him know there is a problem. You are more important to your spouse than the other woman. My point, however, is this guy found it necessary to lie because he had a small unit. Most women would not have been so accommodating and would have pitched a fit for him lying about it. Asking for drama in a situation is not a good avenue to take and a guy hoping for a mercy fuck is so unappealing. If he had used some humor and was honest about his size he might have won the woman over with his charm and the unit size would have been secondary. Blatantly lying about a crucial element as to the size of your unit is taking your life into you own hands gentlemen. Be honest because they are going to find out the facts sooner or later.

Mr. Empty Pants...

The first half a dozen times when you play you may encounter a couple of very common problems. You are so worried about making a good impression, handling the situation eloquently, making sure you wife is happy and secure, impressing the other woman, making points with the other man and all these side issues have made you Mr. Empty Pants. You are so distracted that your dick won't cooperate. I know many of you are thinking, "No possible way that's going to happen to me. I'm going to have a rock solid hard-on that won't stop." Well, maybe you will be one of the lucky ones and pull it off effortlessly the first time around. The majority of you are going to have issues. Don't beat yourself up about it and when it happens, make light of it with humor and turn the focus to oral.

I shouldn't have to remind people of this but I will anyway. Please remember that alcohol can impede a nice hard on. Too much alcohol is very likely to make you Mr. Empty Pants, so curb it for the evening.

Many men young and old like to take a safety measure, so they don't have to think about Mr. Empty Pants. That is the use of sexual enhancing medications. This gives a guy the extra security that, should the brain let him down; the meds will back him up. I have even seen this fail on occasion, so nothing is guaranteed.

Another form of Mr. Empty Pants is for a guy to ejaculate too quickly in the play session. This only happened once to me and I think it surprised the guy too. We had just arrived at our local favorite swing club and started playing with this couple in their late 40's. The night was very young and we had been playing with them about 10 minutes and while I was doing a hand job with this guy he came suddenly. Well, needless to say I saw them packing up their things about 20 minutes later and leaving the club. It's not uncommon for the evening to be finished when the male half comes. Especially if he is 35 plus in age and has a long turn around period or no turn around period. This is one reason the majority of men wait until late in the evening after they have played with many women before they finally decided to cum. Gentlemen, if this happens to you then you need to be prepared with your wife on a plan of action. Do you go off by yourself and chat with others while she continues to play? Does she find a good stopping point and exit with you for the evening? This is something that you have to decide on ahead of time.

Rejection...

Something in the Lifestyle that you need to get used to is rejection. If you have a hard time dealing with rejection then you are going to have a hard time in the Lifestyle. You can't please everyone and each person has their own unique set of standards that they are looking for in a playmate. It's not always appearance if you get turned down. Many people want to know why they are being rejected and I think that's asking for trouble. Does it really matter? Ultimately, it does not. Whatever the other person feels it's right for them and you most likely won't view it the same as them. Whatever they decide on, you are going to have to accept and not care why they turned you down. One person may think you are too fat and the next person will tell you that you are too thin, when in reality you are HWP (height weight proportionate). It's their reality and their perspective and it doesn't matter what you think you are, but what is their perception of you. Consequently, no one is right or wrong when making a decision to turn someone down. Plus, don't ask why, because that's just plain tacky and you aren't going to agree with them on their reasoning, so don't even go there.

Another very important thing that people seem to forget (which is very important) is the fact that most people you encounter in the Lifestyle don't know the "real" you. In reality, it takes months if not years to truly know a person and call him a friend. When people in the Lifestyle reject you and you have only just met, then they are only rejecting their "image" of you. They aren't rejecting the "real" you. If they took the time to get to know you over months it might have a different ending, but that's not how decisions are made in the Lifestyle. People have to weed out the people they don't want to play with and leave time for those that do meet their criteria. Plus, there are no right and wrong standards. Everyone has their right to like and desire what they will and if you don't fit, then don't stress on it and move on. It's that simple.

Hygiene

Don't think you guys you get off so easy here! Most men forget there are aspects under normal circumstances that can be ignored, but not when it comes to playing with strangers. Your wife will overlook things, but we female playmates won't. Men please remember to trim your nose hairs! Obviously, a close shave is also in order, since none of the women want rug burns on their pussies! I have had a few guys with thick stubble who told me they shaved that morning but didn't shave again when getting ready for the party that evening. You will need to trim your package up too. Stop arguing about it and just do it. Stand over the toilet and comb out your pubic hair to get rid of those loose ones. Take a pair of scissors and trim your hair down to about an inch long. The girls usually don't like a whole bunch of hair down there. If you are bold enough, you might even use a razor in the shower and really trim up the patch down there (or have your wife do it). Most of the ladies don't care for a lot of body hair on guys. One big turn off for most of us is the gorilla look, which is a man having a lot of hair on his back and buttocks. I would highly suggest going to a spa and having a waxing done and take off some of that hair. Yes, it's painful but it will last much longer than shaving it off. Once you are trimmed up the next worry is exfoliation. You must buff your skin from head to toe to get rid of those bumps. You need your skin to be smooth and don't forget the moisturizer once out of the shower.

An often overlooked area on men is the fingernails and toenails. Please clean and trim them up. It's much easier for a guy just to go get an appointment at the local hair salon with the nail technician and have a pedicure done. Guys, they massage your feet and use a sandstone on your heel calluses to make your feet smooth. Then they will trim the nails and put on a coat of clear polish. Guy's feet can be so ugly! Don't forget to use the deodorant and just a little splash of cologne. Don't use much cologne, because once you start sweating during playing, it's going to reek and rub off on your playmates. Yuck! Finally, floss your teeth, brush and gargle... and pocket the breath mints as needed.

Self Control...

Many men worry about their self control in a room full of naked people. Well, remember your wife is with you so that in itself is going to give you lots of self control. The self control most people worry about is the problem with premature ejaculation. I'm sure it happens to men on occasion. I have never run into it. I see the opposite happening more often. Men's anxiety levels are so high that their erection goes south. They can't seem to maintain an erection for a good period of time. Being in a room with others can be overwhelming and don't beat yourself up if the first few times you have some problems. It's even hard for many men to relax enough with someone new and be able to cum. It may take two or three encounters with the same people before a man is able to ejaculate with the other woman. That is a big factor and you need to be aware of this potential.

Let's talk dirty...

Many guys love to talk dirty to the ladies. My husband is definitely one of those guys! The only thing you have to be careful about is how far to take the nasty talk. Not all women like all dirty talk. The easiest thing to do is ask the lady what she likes.

If you aren't comfortable being that forward then as you are playing whisper in her ear questions like "Do you like to be called a bitch?" She will let you know. I for one don't like to be called names. They are too derogatory for me and they just piss me off when I hear them. There are women, however, that love being called names and you can even call them the "C" word and get away with it. Not only talking dirty can be an issue but talking in general can be a major issue. My husband loves to ask questions and make dirty statements in sex. I love to hear it, but I have a very hard time responding back verbally. For me to be in the throes of passion and have to form a sentence that makes any sense takes me out of the situation. So for me to do a lot of talking is very uncommon. Then again there are women that talk too much and you just want to shut them up. Everyone has their own way of doing things and there is no right or wrong way of doing it. You just have to find people that are compatible to your standards.

DOIN ONE FOR THE TEAM

Chapter Seven

MIND GAMES

Sometimes, friendship versus just playmates, gives many people more comfort with moral issues, when dealing with the reality of swinging.

One fact we all have to face and that is we are human. With that there is always going to be some mind games involved in activities that are new and different. I'm not trained in psychology but what I have observed over the years seems to be very consistent in the swing community. One of the largest personal mind games that swingers have to play is the justification in their heads (and their moral values) of whether to gear their playing towards friendship or just playmates.

Friendship seems to be a very sought after commodity in the Lifestyle. People say they are looking for friends to entertain in and out of the bedroom and make it a high expectation on their profiles. That criterion makes it even more difficult to find playmates, because not only do they have to be attractive to you but also carry qualities that you find important that equate to friends. That's asking for a lot. Many people look for this quality over quantity, but I have to remind you not to get disappointed if your search is extensive and play sessions few. Why do people add this extra element to their criteria of needing friends? Well, there are many reasons. Many people can't relax sexually around someone, unless they know them really well. To know someone well, means they are a friend, because you have allowed them the time and the depth of contact to reach a level of trust among yourselves to expose the real you. One of the other reasons, is that they need mental "justification" to be doing the swinging morally and feel that with friends' means it has extra meaning and not such a superficially taboo and lustful act. It seems to make many people much more comfortable when they have a caring relationship with the other playmates. This is important to many people. These swingers want friends that do everything with them and even take it so far as to form an emotional bond with the other couple. Obviously, this can be dangerous if all parties aren't on the same page for their feelings and require extremely mature attitudes in handling the situation.

The other type of Swingers, really don't want to be friends. This is the other side of the spectrum and the two are so opposite that they really have a hard time understanding the other type. Many people only want play buddies. My husband and I, happen to fall into this category. We have a deep loving relationship along with many vanilla friends and simply don't have the extra time to cultivate many friends in the swing world. We usually don't do things outside the bedroom with our playmates. Friendship is not usually a consideration in the equation. People that think like us, it usually doesn't matter to them what the person does for a living or how successful they may be or what type of house or car they drive. In other words, to get right down to it they don't care what your favorite color is because they just want to play with you. Obviously, with these types of relationships it's much easier to find playmates, because you have fewer criterions. You don't have to be "friend" material in their book. It's hard enough to find people attractive to you to play with, but to add another layer of being friendship material really adds complications to the equation. This is the only way many people will consider swinging is to always have the people to be friends. Personally, I have never understood it because one of the reasons we got into the Lifestyle was for variety. If you do the same friends over and over then where is the variety? It's always the same people. Whenever people in the Lifestyle happened to become our friends they eventually drop off our list to have sex with, because it can become boring to us. Knowing what to expect from the person takes away that added surprise and thrill we get with being with someone new. So, everyone has to find their own comfort zone and what thrills them. For some it's the new and for others it's the established.

Another difference that divides these two groups is the intimacy factor. One group enjoys intimacy with others and the other group can be repelled by the intimacy. You have to discover which is comfortable for you and your spouse. My comfort is sharing intimacy with my spouse, but with no one else. My emotional side is saved for him and I only share my physical side with others. It's this division of the two that many times separates couples into the two categories. Many people cannot separate the physical from the emotional and consequently need the friendship route to enjoy the Lifestyle. Both ways are unique and satisfying in their own ways along with both having their down sides. So, you must decide what fits your needs.

Sometimes, friendship versus just playmates, gives many people more comfort with moral issues when dealing with the reality of swinging. This can be a major hurdle for some people when trying to make that final decision to enter into the Lifestyle. Ultimately, no one else can make the decision for you and you have to decide for yourself what are good and bad morals. My own opinion is anything that adults can do together that shows affection and caring for a fellow human being is not a bad thing. If it brings comfort and enjoyment it's a good thing. Showing affection towards others and enjoying good times with them is not a bad thing in my book, no matter how you look at it. If there are religious guidelines that are holding you back then you have to evaluate what the supreme power in the universe sees when it comes to affection towards others. Since swingers look at the sex act as just sex and doesn't include love, then its not the same marital sex that two people that love each other have. It's a different type sex that is more animalistic in nature and the embodiment of love and marriage are a separate type of sex. Everyone knows that making love to your spouse is different from fucking an almost total stranger. So, keep in mind that swinging sex is recreational sex and not what you have with your spouse.

One of the key issues when dealing with the Lifestyle is what outsiders (vanilla friends) are going to think about your new activities. Some people share this new adventure with vanilla friends and family and others choose to keep it completely private for various reasons. Let's face it; there are many people out there that will judge you in a negative way due to your sexual activity. I think many do judge you based on their upbringing, their moral values from birth and the total inability to conceptualize such sexual freedom. Obviously, many people that know absolutely nothing about the Lifestyle will jump to the conclusion that it's a free for all with no boundaries and no guidelines. They are shocked to hear that many times you can go to a Lifestyle party and find no one to play with and leave even though others are in front of you naked and screwing their brains out. Many people also will judge you based on their religious beliefs that marriage is sacred and sharing your spouse with another is "going to hell" territory. I'm at a loss as to why there is such major judgment on what other adults do in their personal life. My own viewpoint is that any two humans that engage in an activity that is loving towards others and freely expresses a positive caring attitude is not likely to be a negative in the eyes of my supreme being. That is my own opinion, however, such as it is. I know between myself and the supreme power that the engagement of an enjoyable activity between two adults is not going to put me on the black list and make me go to the end of the line when it comes to my own judgment day. Showing compassion and caring towards others in a sexual act is not something that is a negative. Both people feel great coming out of the experience and each has gained a better understanding of what is truly important in life - how you treat other people. Now, if you enter the Lifestyle with the attitude that you are going to use and abuse people that is totally different and not only will that likely get you black marks on our report card, but also word will get around in the Lifestyle community and you won't get many repeat playmates. So, if you are having a battle between your brain and your heart on this issue then listen to your heart in what is right between you and your inner self. Go with what is comfortable and acceptable to your own voice.

Chapter Eight

SEXUAL ORIENTATION

Straight males are a minority, because most women in the Lifestyle are bisexual and bi-curious.

One of the key factors that everyone stays cognizant of when choosing potential playmates is sexual orientation. This is also an area that has many interpretations of just what the labels mean. Everyone has their own definition. The three main orientations are straight, bi (bisexual) and bi-curious. There are some others like bi-comfortable but we are going to stick with the three main orientations.

Straight...

There is no doubt that the majority of men in the Lifestyle are straight and the majority of women are bi or at least bi-curious. It can be very difficult for straight people wanting to find other straight people because it is the one real minority. People attribute this to many different reasons, but my own reason for the majority of women being bi oriented is that the Lifestyle itself is a non-traditional adventurous avenue for people to take, so it isn't a huge stretch for them to also seek a non-traditional orientation. We all can get vanilla sex as straight individuals and that is the most common relationship type sex. The experimentation in the Lifestyle also leads to experimentation in sexual orientation. It is very acceptable for women to play with other women, yet it hasn't reached the same for men to be bi or bi-curious. With women it is acceptable to be bi and the judgmental attitudes many times can come when they find out you are a straight female. Straight females are a minority, because most women in the Lifestyle are bisexual or bi-curious.

Straight females are looked at as traditional and limited in their play. They have a narrow corridor of options compared to the bi and bi-curious females. Just what is a straight female? I personally think a straight female is one that has no intention or desire to be physical with another woman. This includes kissing, caressing, touching and all sensuous oriented affection. They strictly want to touch, kiss, caress and play with men only. With this said, I have run into straight women (at least they label themselves straight on their websites) that will kiss another woman and or caress her breasts and even as much as fondle her breasts. Some straight women have even allowed me to go down on them orally, which to me just doesn't reflect being straight. There is also a small minority of bi women that label themselves on their websites as straight, but only do so because they don't want women to think they will play with all women or feel obligated to play with women. As you can see, being labeled straight doesn't always mean no physical contact with other women. This is why it's very important to ask a straight woman when you are first corresponding to find out what are their limitations. Everyone will have their own guidelines.

Straight men are much easier to classify because it means they don't desire any physical sexual contact with other men. There are two types of straight men. There are the homophobes, that freak when another guys cock brushes against them or if they're in close proximity. Thankfully, these homophobes are very rare and frankly I think they just haven't evolved as men yet, but then that's my own personal opinion. Most straight men in the Lifestyle are not homophobic and don't desire sexual contact with other men, but it also doesn't bother them to be close to another cock. If two men are in a threesome with a female and they are double teaming her and one guy's cock is in her vagina and the other guy is in her ass, each guy has to be able to withstand close contact and even accidental touching without it affecting them. There are even some men that label themselves as straight that would allow a bi-guy to touch them or give them a blow job.

Bi-Curious...

People that are bi-curious should simply be people that are curious about bisexual play. Once they experience bi-play then they should move to being straight or bi. People can't be curious forever. You see people labeling themselves as bi-curious year after year. Come on people, once you have experimented in this area you either know you are bi or not. Unfortunately, many people don't like to be committed to anything, so bi-curious is not straight or bi and seems the vague way out. Many people that I run into that are labeled forever as bi-curious have said they do so because they want the option of *not* playing with the same sex. They don't want others thinking that just because you are a bi female that you will play with all females. They state they are "bi-situational" and must be attracted to you. No kidding people! Everyone is "sex situational" and needs to be attracted to the other person. Just because you are bi doesn't mean you will play with all bi people just like those with a straight orientation are not going to play with every straight person. That kind of thinking is just absurd.

Bisexual...

The majority of females are bi-oriented in the Lifestyle. Bisexual means you play with both sexes. Now, many people think you have to like men more than women or women more than men and they have all sorts of definitions of what they think a bi-person should be. Bi women, like straight and bi curious women have their limitations too. There are stereotypes of bi women that need to be discussed. Many people think if you are bi then you will play with anything on two feet. People think you are very promiscuous and are so sexual that you don't have limitations like other orientations. This is simply not true. Everyone has limitations and guidelines and theses are things you must find out before playing with others. Some bi women will not go down on women and even some bi women judge them as not bi. Not every straight woman gives blow jobs, so does that keep her from being classified as straight? Huh?

Another misconception about bi women is that men think they are more into women than men. Now, there may be some bi women that fit this case but they don't seem to be the majority that I have encountered. Most bi women are married to men and men come first and women are second. I personally feel if I preferred women I would be a lesbian instead of being bi. This is my own interpretation. Many bi women feel that if another bi woman won't eat pussy that she really isn't bi. Well, I don't follow this line of thinking. I think everyone has their own limitations of what they like.

Many people go into the Lifestyle for sex and not emotional relationships. Emotional relationships can be done in the vanilla world and its sex that sets the Lifestyle apart from the traditional world. I see being bi in the Lifestyle as strictly desiring sex with males and females and not desiring emotional relationships with both. I personally enjoy playing with males and females (although I prefer males) but I could never fall in love with a female and have a "relationship" with her. I am only able to do that with a man.

Unfortunately, people are still judgmental and bisexual men in the Lifestyle are the least accepted by the majority. There are two types of bi men that I have encountered and they are those that will do only oral with other men and those that do everything including penetration. Now, do men that enjoy penetration with just their wife through butt plugs and strap-ons deem themselves as bi? No. I know several men that enjoy having their wife put on a strap on and using it on them, but they have no desire to have a real guy do the deed. They label themselves as straight because they have no desire to play with men. What you do just between you and your wife doesn't count.

Chapter Nine

SIGN ME UP

If you want people to take you serious then you are going to have to pay for a membership on a swing website.

You've discussed it with your partner and now have decided to take the next step, to see if the Lifestyle is truly something for both of you. Believe me, not everyone knows for sure up front and it takes some small steps in the beginning to inch towards a decision on what you would like to experience. Let's face it, fantasy is different from reality. No one really knows how they will react in any given situation until they are in that situation for the first time. You might think you know how you will react, but in reality you don't know until you encounter it.

The very first step is to sign up on a website that caters to Swingers. There are hundreds of them. I have my favorites and after trying about a dozen different sites I pretty much settled for one major site that we are a lifetime member. Just this one site when I sign on, shows how many other people are currently on line. The average is around 6000 people on line across the country. Just in one week there have been 10,000 new members join the site. Obviously, this does not account for all the members not on line at that given moment. Some of the sites are worldwide, so if you travel a lot you can search for whatever country you happen to be visiting. Everyone has their own favorite site and I'm sure mine are different from others. My husband happens to be over 50 years old, so there is one site which is an absolutely great site but it really caters to the younger crowd below 35, so we don't get much email on that site.

Each site requires the same things from you. You make a profile as a single or a couple based on several factors. They will ask both your sexual orientation, your age and your weight and you fill out a lengthy profile telling what you are like, what you are looking for and your fantasies. I found when I filled out several different sites, I could just cut and paste my responses from other sites, so I didn't have to take the time to start from scratch on each sites initial questions. They will ask you to upload pictures of both of you and depending on whether they are "G" rated or "X" rated they can be flagged as "private" pictures, where you control who sees those pictures. If you want another couple to see your private pictures then different sites have different guidelines, but there is always some method on the site to click onto that person's profile which "allows" them to see your private pictures. Many people feel more secure with most of their pictures in private, but also be aware that this will lower the number of people that will contact you. When people are surfing the site to see who is on-line in their area (usually governed by zip code) then those with pictures will get responses faster than those that don't post a picture.

Many websites have different levels of membership and those that sign up for "free" status are the lowest and don't' get all the viewing perks. Real players many times don't take them that seriously. If you want people to take you seriously then you are going to have to pay for a membership on a swing website. I like the lifetime memberships because you never have to worry about it again and everyone knows you are a serious player if you are going to pay top dollar for you membership on that site.

Another important factor is certifications on a site. Different sites call it different things, but the bottom line of it is that other members of the website that you have played with can write a certification for you that it's posted on your profile for all to read. This shows two things - what they thought of you and that you are real and not fake. You always have the option to reject anyone's certification that they may write for you, so if you didn't hit it off with a couple don't think that they can write something negative and you not have control of what is reflected on your profile.

One thing many of the larger sites give you are the forums. This is an area you can bring up a question and let everyone on the website post comments to it. Reading the forums is a great way to learn about swinging and going into their history files will bring many hours of informative reading.

Let's go over a few of the basic elements of a website membership and what needs to be considered when setting up a profile for the entire universe to view.

Handle

Everyone has a handle (fake name) on these websites. I would suggest you come up with something that is unique to yourselves and has some personal meaning. Then as you develop other profiles on other websites always use the same handle and same passwords, so you never have to second guess each site. We choose the handle Simbaxxx. Simba, has a personal meaning to my husband and I and the "xxx" just seemed appropriate. Sites allow alpha and numeric characters so the combinations are endless.

Orientation

Different sites call it different things but you first choose if you are a single person or a couple. Then you must decide what sexual orientation each of you are in the Lifestyle. Not everyone has the same descriptions. The common ones are, straight, bi-curious and bisexual. There are others that may have bi-comfortable but they aren't as prevalent a description. Now if you aren't sure what you are then default to what you think you are and as you experiment you can always change your orientation later.

Height, Weight and Age

Okay here are some very sensitive points that you need to decide how you are going to address. There are advocates of absolute truth. There are also advocates of telling what you look like not what reality dealt you. Most people that see 160 lbs on a woman will think she is fat. But, if that woman is 5' 8" then that's average weight, but people tend to not take that into consideration. You have to decide how you are going to present yourself. My husband and I easily look 10 years younger than our actual ages. I did an experiment once and put our actual ages on our profiles and tracked the contacts. Then I switched the ages to reflect what we really looked like in person (what others have told us). You wouldn't believe the difference between the amounts of inquiries we received. There are several breaking points on ages, but in general they are 30, 40 and 50 years of age. People have cut offs set in their head of below each of one of those decades. It's a shame that people have their cut off ages but some people I guess can't handle that they are fucking someone that is the same age as their parents. HA!!! I have to admit that I got a bit rebellious in my profiles and put down that I was 18 years old and my husband was 99 years old once. That way no matter what age bracket they searched we would pop up in their age bracket. More importantly, however, they could see that we were obviously grossly lying on our ages and our profiles made fun of it. My tag line was "Doesn't he look great for 99!!!" I stated in my profile that if you must know our real ages then just ask. No one asked. This truly amazes me because people make such a stink about "Not wanting anyone over 40" or "Must be between 35 and 45" etc. Think about it - when it comes right down to it, does their age really matter? Doesn't it tend to be more about how a person looks that matters? Age is just relative because many people don't look their age. If someone looks attractive to you then their age would seem irrelevant for most people.

Tag Line

Every profile has a tag line. It's that one sentence that people view during a search that gives them a tidbit of information about you can grab their attention. Tag lines should be rotated and changed every couple weeks to keep them fresh. I've seen profiles stay the same for years. Come up with a snappy attention grabber line and use it as your tag line. I try to never repeat my tag lines, but over the years it has become hard to invent something new and different.

Describe yourselves

Somewhere in the profile it is going to ask you to describe yourself. Obviously you want to capture the positive aspects of you and your spouse, so talk about what you want to reveal to other people reading your profile. The following is an example of our own description on one of the websites.

She is beautiful with 38D's and stays fit with working out and outdoor activities. She is very lighthearted and has a fantastic sense of humor. The more aggressive you are the more aggressive she will get both with males and females. She loves cocks, strap-ons and all toys and her oral skills on men and women are terrific!!!

He is very handsome, 6'4" lean and muscular. He is very direct and loves to talk dirty with the ladies.... and the best sense of humor. Ladies he will make you walk away weak kneed after a session with his tongue and his well hung unit...LOL!

You can put as much or as little into the profile, but remember that too little makes you look less serious. Both are not good things.

Usually another section of a profile will ask you to explain what you are looking for. Here is our description of what we are looking for on one of our websites.

We enjoy meeting where we have the option to play on premise if things go well. We generally set up meetings with new couples at clubs or at private house parties. We can have a few drinks at the club or party and if things click ...let's play!

Couples... we are looking for "playmates". However, should friendship happen we certainly will cultivate it but friendship takes time so sex will come first.

She loves riding a cock, but also likes the added eroticism of female play WITH her cock if it's available.

Our favorite is to "double team" a woman. The two of us will work together and "consume" a female until the woman is totally exhausted.

*** SORRY- WE ARE NOT LOOKING FOR SINGLE MALES AND CONDOMS ARE A MUST***

Another part of the profile will be an area that you can write out your fantasies. Many people go to great lengths to actually list their fantasies, but there is also an equal number of people that dismiss it to "too many to mention so ask us when we meet" sort of remark on the respective area.

Sometimes there is an added space for any additional comments and I usually like to set apart the fact that we always use condoms and state this on the profile.

Photos

One of the major influences on whether you will receive inquires is your photos. If you are very timid and need lots of discreetness then take photos that exclude your head. Just include your body in the photo and it can be "G" rated photo. Different websites have different rules and some of them don't allow the default photo to show frontal nudity. Butt shots always get a lot of response along with breast shots. Sorry ladies, but since most of the surfing on these sites is done by the male, then most profiles gear their default pictures to capture the male's attention. Don't forget to put up a few photos of the male because she needs to approve the profile too, if there is going to be any potential contact.

The photo on the front cover of this book is one of our many profile default photos. It shows a sexy attitude and displays enough to capture what I look like and make a judgment on possible interest. Your pictures are your best friend when it comes to people wanting to make contact. It depends on how bold you want to be in your statement with your default picture and obviously if you aren't afraid of putting your face out there then you will get even more responses. You have to decide how bold you will be with your pictures.

As far as the private pictures are concerned, you can be "x" rated, but because of the new laws many sites limit crotch shots and true explicit sex photos. We happened to stay away from explicit pictures such as those, because we don't happen to find them classy. We have one nude photo of myself, but it shows me standing there nude and doesn't show close ups of my genitalia. I just happen to think close up shots of your genitals is unnecessary and a bit tasteless. That's what is great about the Lifestyle, the variety of approaches.

Once you have your profile finished and pictures loaded (many times a 24 hour approval process) then you are ready to start making some contacts. Now you have two approaches you can take in starting out in the Lifestyle. You can get your feet wet by going to a club and witnessing the happenings in a club to see if you would feel comfortable engaging in such activities or meeting one on one with another couple and scoping them out in hopes to further explore your options with them.

My favorite option for Newbies, which we followed ourselves when starting out in the Lifestyle, was to attend a club. Now at first you may think there is no way you would go to a club. Please listen to my reasons for doing so, before you cast judgment. One of the scariest parts of encountering this new Lifestyle is being in the "spot light". No one new wants to be put on the spot or be the center of attention when just starting out. Most Newbies want to fade into the background and be a shadow. Now, how can you do that if you are meeting just one on one with another couple? There is no place to hide and you are put on the spot by the other couple directly asking you questions that you may at first not feel comfortable answering. If you go to a club where there are 100 people, then you can get lost in the crowd and no one will ever notice that you didn't participate or get naked. In a crowd you can go undetected and observe the happenings of swingers without being put on the spot to participate. Many of the clubs allow people to mill around the bar and dance floor area and then also casually walk around the play areas and observed while you are still fully clothed. What a hot idea for those that don't yet know how far they want to go in the Lifestyle than walk around fully clothed watching others completely naked and playing! Usually at the clubs, the bar and dance floor area people are fully clothed and it just seems like a really sexy clientele of a vanilla bar that most people encounter. Granted there may be a few women who fondle each other or do things that don't happen at normal bars but for the most part the bar/dance floor area of a swing club is pretty tame compared to the hidden play areas that are usually behind the scenes.

Emails...

Obviously, one of the biggest first steps is finding another couple on a website that you want to contact. Don't write some long diatribe that takes forever for someone to read. That's why you put so much effort and thought in writing your profile, so all the pertinent information is already there. Just write a few sentences and tell them BOTH what drew you to their profile. Compliment them and ask them to read your profile to see if they have interest. I always think it's a good thing to always open your private pictures for people you are sending emails. There are a huge percentage of people that keep all their pictures under private so you have nothing to look at when you receive an email. Now, how can you tell if you are interested in them if you can't see what they look like. I have just never understood that concept. If you contact someone then open up your pictures to them.

Most people don't want a whole lot of emails dragging back and forth, so after two or three then suggest a phone call. Calling verifies they are real and ask to call them when they are both available and can be on the line together. It's always good to talk to both, so there are no misunderstandings on what people are looking for and expect. Too many times we have been in situations where the wife didn't know anything about us and she also was not as bisexual as the husband led us to believe in our earlier conversations. Sometimes the bisexual play is wishful thinking on his part and you have to sift through to the truth. The only way that will happen is to speak to both. Once you feel that all of you are attracted then suggest you meet for drinks somewhere or meet at a local swing club for drinks. As you become more experienced you will know how much contact you need prior to setting up a meeting. In the beginning, you are unsure of things and tend to be overly cautious. As time moves on, you will be able to judge much more quickly and may not even need a phone call and just tell them you are going to the local swing club on a given night and if they would like to meet you then you would be happy to see them there. That way there is no pressure on anyone and there are always plenty of people to meet at a club.

Recognizing Flakes and Fakes...

Newbies in the Lifestyle are always surprised when they discover that someone isn't real or turns out to be a flake. Flakes are those that will pursue you and then all of a sudden disappear. You make appointments with them and they don't show up or every time you suggest meeting they always have an excuse. After about three tries we write people off if they can't seem to meet us. We tell them the ball is in their court and to contact us when they are available. Up until that point, they were hot and heavy in their emails and phone calls. Many times it turns out these Flakes are truly Fakes. There are several types of Fakes that you should be aware of.

The picture collectors are those males that want the power of having your picture. They are always hounding you to email copies of your pictures to them. Every few weeks they ask if you have any new pictures. I made it our policy to tell people we don't email pictures. If they want to see us then look at the pictures on our website profile and that should suffice. Many of them, however, use the excuse that their membership is of a lower status (such as free) and they can't view our pictures. When this happens I just tell them to invest in a membership because otherwise people won't take you seriously.

There are verbal sex fakers that are men who usually get the female on the phone under false pretense to just talk dirty. If this is your thing, that's fine. go right ahead because you will find plenty of players in this area. I refuse to do sex talk on the phone with anyone and finally had to make a policy that I would only talk to the wife because men kept tricking me to get on the phone and then turn the conversation to sex talk as he masturbates. That is just not appealing to me.

There are some profiles that say they are bisexual single females and after awhile your conversations with them (usually through your IM's and emails) just doesn't seem quite right. There are certain things females will not talk about and they phrase their sentences differently from males. Single females that turn your IM conversation to crotch descriptions and fantasy details are a red flag warning that it might be a male on the other end. They usually don't have the smooth etiquette and fine language the females have in their descriptions and sentence structures. It's a dead giveaway when they start being blunt, direct and vulgar with their questions and descriptions.

There are some people that are classified as the "wanna be's". They sound promising and your endless emails with them never seem to materialize. Many times this can be just a cheating husband on the other side playing out his fantasies through emails. Some cheaters will go as far as to set up a meeting and then when they arrive, the wife isn't with them. They state that they just wanted to keep the appointment with you. This is another big warning flag as a cheater. If both aren't there, then cancel the meeting until both can make it in the future. No one wants to play with a cheater, and neither do you want to enable a cheater to cheat, so don't let it go any further when you sense a cheater.

You will encounter many fakers out there so keep your radar up and tuned into the red flag warnings. If your gut instinct tells you something smells fishy, then it most likely is fishy. It will be time to cut your losses and move on to another hot prospect, because there are a lot of them out there for the picking.

Chapter Ten

OUR FIRST PLAY DATE

Always keep other people's rules in mind and respect their boundaries.

Okay you have been emailing and IMing back and forth with a couple (or a single) and you've decided to meet. One of the scariest times is that very first date with another Swinger. I would suggest you find someone that is not in the same boat, so you can be directed by someone that has more experience. They don't have to be very experienced, but don't choose someone else that is on their first date too. You have to decide where you would be the most comfortable in meeting others. Some people like to go have drinks and socialize. They tell the other couple they don't play on the first date and must be up front about this information. There are many people (like us) that won't go out with people that won't play on the first date if everything goes well. Dinner is another alternative, but you must remember that if you don't hit it off well, you are stuck in the middle of having dinner with them; whereas, if it's just drinks after one round you can get up and leave.

Whether you decide to meet at a normal bar, restaurant or a swing club the actual initial meeting will generally follow about the same course. Unfortunately, many people are too afraid to approach the core of the discussion and spend way too long on talking about personal vanilla issues. Nothing is wrong with normal vanilla chit chat but within the first 20 minutes try to get around to asking some swing oriented topics that will get them to open up. Here are a few questions that should help to know them better.

- How long have you been in the Lifestyle?
- How did you get into the Lifestyle? Who's idea?
- Have you made many friends?
- Where do you prefer to play?
- What is one of funniest things that has happened during playing?

The last question is to help lighten the tone. Everyone knows things can happen during sex and it's to be fun. We all have encountered someone who has passed gas or made some unusual sounds or got their earring caught in someone's hair or started their period during play, etc. Laugh about things that potentially could embarrass you. We all have those fears. It's better to get them out in the open than let them hang over you as worries.

As people talk about themselves things always become more relaxing. It's also easier with these topics to move the discussion toward a more erotic tone if it's warranted. If you find that you really like the couple find a way to compliment them during your discussion. If they are into you they will return the favor at some point during the discussion letting you know they like you too. You aren't going to get many compliments from people that don't have any intentions of playing with you. Great communication is important in swinging and especially with your spouse. At some point, both of you have to discuss (away from your date) how you feel about the new potential playmates. My husband and I had sign language between us that would convey different things and this way we knew (without the other couple knowing) how each of us felt about the situation. Nothing is more embarrassing than your spouse going full speed ahead when you are ready to run in the opposite direction. You need to go into meeting couples with some concrete guidelines and stick to them. It takes the stress level down knowing that you both have decided you will not play on the first date or that you will only soft swap. On the first date, it's easiest just to be up front that you want to go home and discuss things further and that you will be in contact with the couple. You'll want to take things slow if you are unsure.

What if you both give each other the signal and you want to play that night? Ask the couple if they have plans for later and that you would like to invite them over to your house, or back to the playrooms at the club or hotel room (whichever the case may be) for some fun activities if they are interested. The easiest line when at a club is to tell a couple that you have great interest in them and that you are going to take a walk through the playrooms to see if anything is going on and ask would they like to join you. If they have any level of interest in playing with you, then they will make it clear. Either they will join you or they may tell you they have interest, too, but aren't ready just at the moment and will catch up with you later. The "catch up with you later" line can also be used as a nice put off for not wanting to play by some people, so you have to judge on how the conversation went as to their exact meaning. Not everyone is direct about their interest or lack thereof. If they join you in your walk back to the playrooms, then it's easy to start playing with your own spouse while watching others which sets an erotic tone right away for the other couple.

We bi gals have a bit of an advantage in that we can be more open and touchy feely with each other, which acts as a natural catalyst for playing to begin. I just find it much easier to strike up suggestive conversation with the other female on what she is wearing than with some strange man I've known for less than an hour. Everyone finds their own comfort zone. One of the things that men often do to bond is ask for tips about the other's wife - what excites her and what does she like to do and not do. Men trading insight on their wives, seems to help bond their connection.

Many of you will be unfortunate on the first date to meet a flake (or even get stood up). If you are stood up, don't think you've been singled out because it is prevalent in the Lifestyle. I find it rude and unacceptable, but some people have the nerve to not even call to let you know they aren't going to be able to make it. They just leave you hanging. This is one of the reasons we finally starting meeting people at the swing clubs instead of privately for dinner or drinks because people can't be relied on. At the club, if someone doesn't show up, then there are plenty of other likeminded people there to explore.

Should the people you meet turn into a flake and you don't want to play with them then tell them you don't think you are right for each other and leave it at that. Now, there are people that insist on some explanation and that is a no win situation. Don't do it. It doesn't matter what you say, they won't like it and will try to rebut it. Gracefully bow out that you aren't in the mood right now, or if you have the balls, be bold and tell them you aren't attracted. Personally, I can't tell someone I'm not attracted to them. I don't care who you are and how self assured you are, no one enjoys hearing they are not attractive. I always tell people that I find them interesting (and I really do but just not enough to play with them) but I'm not ready to play right now and I may catch up with them later. Most people accept that subtle reject and don't approach you later in the evening. Other people will be blunt about it, but conceal it by using a term that lends itself to the fact that they have no control over it and it is what it is. They tell you the "chemistry" just isn't there…another subtle statement of just saying they just don't find you attractive.

Maybe during your first date you are lucky and you decide to be bold and play with the new couple you have met. Make sure before you start your foreplay that you have asked each other what is off limits. Some people won't have any limits and others will have too many. These limits will be like no kissing with the tongue, no anal sex, condoms only, same room play, etc. Always keep other people's rules in mind and respect their boundaries. No one will put up with someone trying to push another past their rules. One of the worries I had the first few times we played with others is the timing of the finishing of our play. What if my partner and I finish, before my husband and his partner? Do I stand around and pick my nose at him or do I go off and grab something to eat and drink? Well, there is another alternative which my husband and I prefer and that is for me to go over and join him in his play with the other female. This is easy if both females are bi, but if you are both straight then join in the play and concentrate your efforts on your husband. It could be possible that you sense (or are told) by the other female that she prefers to finish it out with just your husband. This indeed is a bit of a sticky situation because one of our rules is that we don't play separate. We consider ourselves a team. I could set there patiently and watch them finish their session, but after about 10 minutes I'm looking at my watch because that isn't exactly exciting for me. My husband is kind enough to stay aware of this fact and speed up the climax of their play, so everyone is closer to ending their play at the same time. It doesn't bother some people if their spouse continues to play and I've known partners to have to literally wait for a couple hours while they finish. If you don't find that a problem then this won't be an issue for you.

Chapter Eleven

PLAYING WITH SINGLES

Single females are called Unicorns because they seem to be a figment of people's imagination.

Granted, most of this book concentrates on couples in the swing world because that is the majority. There are the single males and females, however, that are listed in the swing sites that enjoy being with couples. There is a certain mindset that needs to be reinforced when it comes to singles.

Male Singles...

Just because you list yourself on a profile on a swing site and you have a cock doesn't make you a swinger. Male singles have a rough road to climb in the swing world because the bad apples leave a bad taste in everyone's mouth and you will have to prove yourself. So, what do the bad apples do?

-Are rude and crude with their approach
to couples.
-Show no class or manners with
their aggressive style.

-Think that the only things people want
to see are cock photos.
-Don't understand the nature of
MFM situations. He is being allowed
to enjoy the loving relationship of the
couple and he is just a nice additive
for fun but not part of their relationship.
-Flake and disappear or are no shows
without warning or explanation.
-Are quick draws out of the holster
with no stamina power.
-Doesn't ask the husband for tips on
the wife because he thinks he can figure
it out on his own. This aspect has to do
with bonding and respect of the
husband more than anything.

Now, some things that a couple needs to remember when dealing with single males is to set back and allow the single male to hang himself on his own. Wait for him to ask you what your wife likes and dislikes and don't volunteer the information. If he doesn't ask then that is a test of his character and you had better beware. Couples also need to remember that that it is much easier for single males to get laid through the vanilla route than the swing world so don't think you are doing them any favors.

Female Singles...

It is just as hard to find good single females as it is good single males. Single females are called Unicorns because they seem to be a figment of people's imagination. Don't get me wrong. There are plenty of single females listed on swing sites, but they are as hard to nail down as a cloud. They also get a bad reputation because of different reasons as the single male. There are few good ones out there but you have to go through a crap load of flakes to find one. By then you wonder if the search was worth it. In the past 3 years, we have encountered two good single females and the rest were drama queens and way too much work. What do Unicorns do that leave a bad taste in your mouth?

-They think the world revolves around them and they flake on you.
-They are scared off easily and think they can handle a situation and can't.
-They don't bond with the wife.
-The Unicorn thinks the husband is going to show her loving and caring affection.
-She thinks she "means" something to the husband when in reality it's just sex.
-Many couples don't want to hear her issues or her boyfriend problems.
-She wants more than the couple is willing to offer.
-She tries to get in between the wife and husband.
-The Unicorn is too emotional and gets too attached.
-They lead people on and then have no follow through.

I do have a few words of advice if you are a single female wanting to get involved in the swing world. Remember that you will always be icing on the cake but never be the cake. Don't expect to be the cake and don't act like you have rights to be the cake. Be more respectful of people's time because the world usually doesn't revolve around you. If you make an appointment, keep it and be on time or make sure you give plenty of warning. It's easy for singles to drop things and run out for a date without lots of notice provided they don't have kids at home. Many couples do have to go to great pains to secure a babysitter and create a time that they are able to have fun. Be considerate of each other's time. Going out meeting others on your own can be scary, so if you don't think you have the balls for it then don't lead people on. That's frustrating and wastes people's time.

Couples, there are a few things to remember when dealing with single females. They get hit on a lot, so it's not like they are sitting home alone every night. Most of them are skittish and you have to approach them slowly and allow them to warm up to you. Don't be pushy!! Unless of course they said they like lots of aggression. As with all your encounters, treat them with respect and consideration. Meeting strangers for the first time can be a scary situation for a single female, so go the extra mile in making her feel secure and safe. Meeting the first time in a public setting is advisable because it provides the most security for them. As with most females, they like to feel like you care for them and it's not just the sex. Well, as we can stay cognizant of this factor, it's a fine line to walk in the fact that swinging is based on the goal of having sex for many and not always the goal of a friendship. Be honest with the Unicorn if you have no intention of involving them in your life and becoming friends.

DOIN ONE FOR THE TEAM

Chapter Twelve

CLUBS AND HOUSE PARTIES

*We enjoy taking walks through the rooms-
watching people play or just stand by the bed
with my husband fondling my breasts.*

After you have played a few times you will develop a preference on the environment that you feel most comfortable in. They all have unique qualities.

Clubs...

When looking for large places to play the easiest route is to look on the websites that you are members and see if they have listings. Out of the hundreds of websites that are available, our favorite usually has around 14 parties advertised under events in Los Angeles. These are large events held in clubs. The clubs are either in a commercial building or the majority of them are in large homes. These homes are not used by anyone to live in, but are strictly used for commercial swing parties only. Usually you have to join the club to be able to attend. All this is done on line and once you pay your membership dues then you find out their location. Then you will also need to pay as you attend each event which is also all handled on line. One of our favorites has a $50 annual membership and a $100 per attended event fee. The clubs held in large mansions usually have a parking attendant and several host/hostess that monitor the evening and their function is to help you in any capacity whether it's giving you a tour of the facility, answering questions, picking up used towels and linens and monitoring play in the club. They do not participate in the play and act solely in a host capacity. Just about all the clubs provide a buffet with catered food and sodas and mixers. If you want alcohol you usually bring it with you. Generally, the reason for the BYOB is due to zoning ordinances and not needing to have a liquor license. Since most large homes and estates are in residential neighborhoods it needs to keep its true nature below the radar. No one wants a commercial swing club in their neighborhood. Normal house parties are different because they are infrequent and small but we are talking about these clubs having parties every Saturday night with lots of cars and foot traffic with 30+ attendees.

Our favorite typical house club is located on the edge of a neighborhood with a commercial building next door with plenty of parking space. You arrive inside and are immediately greeted by the host or hostess. They check to see that you are on their computer list as paid. If you aren't on that list you will be rejected. Most of the clubs don't allow payment at the door because of potential zoning problems. If you forget to make your payment on line, don't think you will be able to pay at the door. Check first on their website for their guidelines. After checking us off the attendee list, they turn us over to another host/hostess that gives a tour of the facility. Our Manor we attend has a huge gourmet kitchen which has catered food displayed. Usually they will have three hot main courses with some cold finger foods. I usually bring my bottle of Merlot and stand in the kitchen for a few minutes with introductions. You know how everyone congregates in the kitchen during a party? Well, a swinger party isn't any different. The huge living room only has a few pieces of furniture up against the walls so the main area is wide open for dancing. Outside on the covered veranda looking over the pool and hot tub, is an outdoor living space with pedestal heaters keeping the Los Angeles cool evenings warm. The bedrooms are very large and have anywhere from 4 to 6 mattresses on platform beds with beautiful sheer curtains that can be drawn between play areas or left open for we exhibitionist. By each bed platform is a dish full of condoms. Any great club will provide condoms for their patrons. No one wants to be in the heat of passion and all of a sudden discover they forgot to bring their condoms or they have run out. We enjoy taking walks through the rooms watching people play and just stand by the bed with my husband fondling my breasts. He usually lifts my blouse and exposes my breasts for all to see and sometimes the players on the bed will ask to touch them. Usually, that's all it takes for us to get asked to join in the fun. Other times, we just enjoy watching and playing with each other and continue on to other parts of the club enjoying the erotic environment. If no one is playing after the first 45 minutes we will usually go get in the hot tub. Seeing two naked people in the hot tub is a hard thing to ignore and it will usually start up some conversations. If all else fails and we haven't meet anyone to play with then we will go play with just each other in one of the open rooms. It never fails that once we are both naked, it takes about ten minutes before there are other naked people in the room playing. Usually others are just waiting for someone to start playing, so they can start the process too. It is not unusual at these large club parties to have a few hundred people attending here in Los Angeles.

House Parties...

House parties are much harder to find and get an invitation to. These are the non commercial parties, put on by individual swingers. About the only way you can get invitations to these small parties is to know someone. House parties are usually anywhere from 3 couples on up. Obviously, the attendance is governed by the size of their home. You would think more people would host parties at their homes, but it does take a home conducive to these types of parties. Some people only invite people they know, but the majority of people also invite people they have never met. You have to be comfortable with strangers in your house. You also need plenty of areas for play and not be afraid of bodily fluids getting on things. God forbid you have a woman invited that squirts. You could have a flood all over furniture if she isn't taking precautions. Unfortunately, people do not take care of other people's homes like their own. I have never understood this inconsiderateness of people and many people won't be invited back if they don't respect a person's home. It is not uncommon for the hosts to forbid play in their master bedroom because that is their personal domain that they only have sex in and don't allow others in this special place. The most inconsiderate thing I've seen is semen filled condoms lying around the house in every place but the trash can. Come on people, don't act like dogs and please be respectful of people's property and treat it like your own. Discard your own waste!

We have attended many small house parties and once we thought we had hit the jackpot. We found out that the couple we had been corresponding with hosted parties about once every two months and they only lived a few blocks from our house. In Los Angeles it invariably takes an hour or more to get to a party because everything is so spread out. To find a local party a few miles away was wonderful for us. When we attended this couple's first party we had not been to but one other house party at the time. In their initial correspondence with us, they asked us a lot of questions and wanted to make sure we were HWP. They didn't want anyone with any extra padding. When we arrived at their house we were surprised that they weren't in the greatest shape. He was packing about 40 extra lbs and she had about 25 extra pounds, but they both thought for some reason they could be extra picky with their invitees. We ended up hoping the parties would get better, but by the 3rd party we attended at their house, we finally dismissed future invites. Several factors were at play. He was a bit of a Thumper attitude and had the body hair of a gorilla. Now this definitely is not the reason we discontinued, but a funny side note is remembering him walking away from me at a party (totally nude) and seeing that he had completely shaved his butt, so there was no hair on it. He followed the outline of his briefs as a guide. The problem was where he had stopped shaving his buns the rest of his hips and legs had a thick carpet of gorilla hair about two inches long. So, just remember if you are going to start a project you need to finish it. Otherwise get the weed whacker out and finish the job.

The other less than desirable aspect about their parties that influenced us the most is they always invited this one couple we didn't like. They were their best Swinger friends. She was in her early thirties with a terrific body, but was an immigrant from one of the Slavic countries with a very loud boisterous mouth that never stopped talking and always belittled her husband. Granted, he was wimpy (and a Thumper) and not attractive to me, but her chatter never stopped. She was exhausting and we couldn't stand listening to her constant dialog and I got tired of always having to dodge him in these very small parties. So the hassles just didn't out weigh the positives.

Another small factor was that the hostess was labeled bi-curious, but from everything this bi-lady could see was that the husband was doing the labeling. She was pretty much straight. When one straight gal is in a party with 4 other couples and all the other ladies are bi what happens? The straight lady becomes a bit of a "cockhogger" and doesn't share. We bi-ladies want cock too and many times it seemed like she was never going to let loose of any of the men. There is no balance in the play when this happens and it can get frustrating if it persists. Now days when it happens, I'll just join in and make it a 3'some, so I can start playing with the guy too..... which is usually my husband. He really enjoys me approaching him from behind and playing with his "boys" while he has a woman mounted doggie style.

When you decide you are up for a small house party just ask the hosts, who is attending. Sometimes they will give you their handle names, so you can look them up on the websites. Others won't give you the list, so just ask how many confirmed attendees they have and are any of them actual friends of theirs. Ask if there is a theme for the evening that you can dress appropriately. When you go to parties always bring your goodie bag and either wear a long coat covering your suggestive outfit or change when you get there. Here is what my own goodie bag has in it.

Bottle of wine
Change of clothes for the trip home including shoes
Various sizes and types of condoms
Rope
Wrist restrains
Blindfold
Whip
Hair clips for the hot tub
Lube
Massage oil
Strap on dildo
Vibrating dildos
Non vibrating dildos
Nipple clamps

Cosmetic items
Wet toilettes
Soapless antibacterial hand cleaner

As you can see I believe in going prepared, although many of these items don't get used. It's really rare that I will pull out a dildo to use on people. Obviously, the clean up factor is a deterrent because it all has to be sanitized between people and afterwards. If you can run anything through the dishwasher that's always a help.

There is one aspect of parties that I need to forewarn you about. Whether it is a club or a house party, the dynamics of a party changes when single men are allowed to attend with their numbers unrestricted. I have never been a person to make assumptions and I tried my best to disprove this impression. "Couples only" parties or "couples only with the numbers of single men being limited" parties are very much the same. The social dynamics and comfortable atmospheres with easy going attitudes are usually the norm.

Early on in swinging we visited a commercial club in Las Vegas that allowed the unlimited attendance of single men. It was seedy and repulsive to me and lacked the dynamics and social intermingling of the couples. I dismissed my initial impressions and after about a year attended a house party that allowed the unlimited attendance of single men. It was exactly the same atmosphere as the Vegas club reflected. If you are looking for an atmosphere to have a gang bang then these parties will certainly be conducive. Don't expect the people at these parties to have the social and cultured manners of the "couples only" parties. Some single men display the refined qualities of warming up to a couple, but too many single guys have the wolf pack mentality. It's that wolf pack atmosphere that can make us lambs jumpy and uncomfortable. I also highly recommend not doing what one single guy did at the party because it's a sure way of not getting to play with a couple. During our conversation with him he revealed the fact that he was married and that he attended swing parties without his wife because "She just isn't into it and stays home with the kids." At that point, there was nothing he could say that would allow me to warm up to him, because all I could think was "You ass….you're cheating on your wife!" Yup! That's really going to win over another female by showing your disrespect towards your wife. He could have sworn up and down that he was swinging with his wife's permission and there would have been no convincing me of that fact.

DOIN ONE FOR THE TEAM

Chapter Thirteen

AFTER ONE YEAR IN THE LIFESTYLE

The first year we were consumed by lustful desires as playtimes approach, but as we gained experience, it became less about the sex and more about the two of us just experiencing new things together.

The most significant change during that first year of playing was our move from soft swap to full swap. Everyone has milestones that are important and after a year you have a good feeling about what you do like and don't like about the Lifestyle. There is a learning curve that first year and you'll encounter things you don't want to repeat.

The initial year is a lot like being a teenager again and experimenting with great lust for the play. You can't wait until the next weekend to get to do some more things and encounter new situations. At some point, the newness will wear off. For us we found it best to never go into a play date with expectations. Our expectations were always wrong in those earlier sessions. Don't build things up in your head over weeks of contact with a couple, only to find they are not able to live up to your fantasy expectations. That's unfair.

One of the nagging concerns that ultimately passes through a Newbie's mind is wondering if their spouse will grow away from them as they encounter fun with others. As you gain experience, you discover after about a year that you and your spouse are closer than ever within your relationship. Obviously, this is provided you had a healthy loving relationship going into the Lifestyle. Experiencing together the intimate fun with others and discussing these inner desires, fears and excitement draws a couple closer. Knowing your spouse's inner desires, wants and needs and helping them to obtain them is a deep intimacy a couple strives for in any close relationship. You are accepting your spouse for who they are and not trying to change them. You love them for their positive and their negative qualities. None of us are perfect and we all have fears and issues that we deal with in life, so we can grow as individuals.

These days, my husband and I, only play about once every two months or so because our life is very full. This is drastically different from the three and four times a month in the beginning. We play to experience different things in life. Just because a play is not optimal, doesn't mean we will pass on the situation like most people. Sometimes we are intrigued by something and knowingly go into a situation that will just be for the shear knowledge of just enjoying the moment, no matter what it may bring After a year of swinging you think you know how a situation will develop because of all the different situations you encounter. The first year we were consumed by lustful desires as playtimes approach, but as we gained experience, it became less about the sex and more about the two of us just experiencing new things together. I especially came to realize that no one will come close to fulfilling me like my husband, so I don't look for intense sexual encounters with others. I just look for fun situations for my husband and I to experience, since everyone else is second best to him in my mind.

During that first year, we had several discussions and phone calls from a guy and his girlfriend that kept trying to get together, but the timing just never worked out. From their pictures on their profile, this guy's Asian girlfriend seemed to have a great figure and although pictures of him were limited, he seemed to be a classy looking guy. Finally, the timing seemed right, so we decided to hook up with them because they were also inviting another couple and three couples are better for us. That's a small party and I admittedly had reservations about it, but my husband said we should go and just enjoy the titillating conversation and see what's up since the guy had been contacting us forever.

The other invited couple that was joining us at the restaurant had only pictures posted of her and she was supposedly known for her great long legs. The only information about him was the statement on their profile that he was Hawaiian. Since we found out about them at the last minute, we decided to wing it because they wanted to meet in the late afternoon. Wow! What a switch from having to meet late at night like most people prefer. We were up for an adventure, so we were to meet them at 4PM at a family restaurant about 30 minutes away. Meeting in a public setting in the afternoon did pose some clothing problems. I had to find something suggestive, but acceptable in the vanilla world. I decided on a short jean skirt and a tight white sweater with a plunging neckline.

We walked in the restaurant and my husband spotted the two couples setting in a booth. It was a booth for four people and not six. How goofy is that! We had even called them earlier from the car saying we were only 10 minutes away because we were caught in traffic. There were plenty of open tables that seated six, so after standing around waiting for permission from a waitress, we all moved over to the larger table. That should have been my first clue that this experience was going to be an unusual one. When they all stood up I got my first full view of everyone, because prior to that I was standing behind my husband. Yikes! The one classy looking guy that had been calling us stood up and he didn't look anything like his picture. He seemed unusually short compared to his photo and about 15 years older. His girlfriend was petite, but not the gazelle in the pictures. She was rough and tough looking and not the small petite person that the picture had implied; although, she was definitely play material for us.

The other couple stood up and greeted us and I wanted to ask, "Where is the Hawaiian?" He was a robust big guy and had some potential, but his personality would definitely make or break it for me. Then his girlfriend stood up. Holy crap! This is a family restaurant and what was she thinking. She had "hourly rental" tattooed across her forehead. Okay, I'm kidding but that's exactly what everyone in the entire restaurant was thinking. She had a micro mini skirt on that had she not been groomed there would have been pubic hair showing. Her long bare legs were stacked on top of 5" high platform shoes. She had a corset top that had her boobies pushed all the way up and I swear I could see part of her right areola peeking out and winking at me. Then she had a sheer short jacket on that matched the corset and it didn't even reach her midriff. Come on people, you don't go out in the vanilla world to a family restaurant dressed like a rental at 4:00PM in the afternoon. Have some class!

I bet money most of you would have high tailed it out of there immediately. We now are intrigued by the bizarreness of the situation. Admittedly, my husband was more inquisitive than I was. We just ordered tea to drink and everyone else was ordering fruity blended daiquiris. The only person that was eating was Ms. Micro Mini and she let it be known she was a strict vegetarian. Her bean burger arrives and it's covered with crispy real bacon. I look over at my husband and gave this huge grin because this situation can't get anymore bizarre as she gleefully bit into her burger.

Mr. Hawaiian is setting on one side of me and keeps chattering away with jokes, obviously fearing those awkward silent moments. Then in the middle of one of his jokes he stops and looks over at me and asks what I'm thinking about because I'm so quiet. I told him exactly what I was thinking at that moment. I said, "I was just admiring the upper arm muscles on her." I nodded over to Ms. Biceps. She looked up at me with a big smile and told me that she did a lot of heavy lifting in her job. She was a nurse who worked in a retirement facility and many patients required movement in beds. Of course that wasn't the type of movement I was thinking about, but I told her, "Well, it certainly shows."

Ms. Micro Mini finishes her burger and asks a direct question, "Well, what are we going to do? We haven't even discussed what we like." I'm wondering to myself how she intends to talk about sex when we are surrounded so closely by other tables full of people in a family restaurant. Whoever picked the restaurant wasn't thinking. I leaned over to my husband and he said, "What do you think?" I said, "It's up to you, Babe. I'll go with whatever you are feeling." I knew my husband would take it further, only because he believes there are no bad experiences. They are all just experiences and you make of it what you want.

The clock was ticking and we all decided it was time to leave. Ms. Micro Mini, asks, "Well, are we going?" The other couple and I said at the same time, "We will follow you to your house." We all parted ways and climbed into our separate cars.

My husband was going to follow them and that meant I needed to make some decisions and let my husband know what my thoughts were about the situation. I told him that I had interest in the two girls, but the two guys didn't turn me on. Although, personality wise I really liked Mr. Hawaiian. He seemed the most "normal" and entertaining of the four of them. I liked his humor. Definitely a nice guy, but as of yet hadn't turned me on, but he still had potential. They said they lived 5 minutes from the restaurant. We are following them and the other couple down the busy four lane street and finally after about 10 minutes, they make a left turn and pull up to a liquor store. Mr. Hawaiian hops out and says his girlfriend needs something. I wanted to say (but bit my tongue), "What besides better taste in daytime clothing?" He promptly returns with his goods (which we never see her use) and makes an immediate U-turn across a busy four lane road. In the meantime, my husband makes reference to the fact that we must have passed four liquor stores on our side of the road a mile back on the main drag we had been traveling on. Finally, we pull up to their house. It takes him a good five minutes wrestling with the padlock he has on the security gate. Maybe it's their high tech security system to keep thieves from stealing their $100,000 worth of vehicles in the driveway. I always find it a little odd when people's cars don't match the home they live in. This was definitely one of those times. She opened an exterior room and we entered right into a bedroom. It had a king size bed and adjacent bathroom. At the time all I cared about was getting out of the 110 degree heat. Ms. Micro Mini, then turned on the stereo and started flipping through their collection of CD's. My husband took my hand and immediately went over to her and started feeling her up. She had no response. So we stopped. Meanwhile Mr. Short and his girlfriend Ms. Biceps are on the bed getting naked and Mr. Hawaiian has disappeared. My husband tries again and starts fondling, Ms. Micro Mini. She leans into him this time, so he continues to undress her.

Mr. Hawaiian, returns to the room and sits down next to the naked couple on the bed. Ms. Micro Mini sets on the edge of the bed as my husband and I caress her. She does have an attractive body and we both get undressed. My husband asks her if she enjoys women and she remarks, "Only certain women and your wife is definitely one of them." That was my clue that she was into some bi-play. I positioned myself between her legs when she announced *the* warning. She was a squirter. I have always heard about squirters but never encountered one so my curiosity was peaked. Would it really be apparent that she was squirting? Come on, how bad can it be? I started going down on her and her boyfriend comes over to the end of the bed to see what we are doing. He reiterates the fact that she is a real squirter and forewarns me that she cums a lot. Of course, I'm thinking how much is a lot? I was too busy to stop playing. All of a sudden, I could tell she was getting close, so I pulled away from her and sat off to her side and just played with her clit with my fingers. Then she came! Whoa! That stream shot out and my husband immediately put his hand over it so it didn't squirt two feet away. I had no idea a woman could do that. There must have been a cup of fluid on the floor. I had always heard that Squirters always look like they are peeing (even though they aren't). This fluid is manufactured by the G-Spot or properly known as the paraurethral gland. Ms. Micro Mini immediately popped up and headed to the bathroom to retrieve a towel to mop up the floor. I wondered why she didn't have a towel handy in the first place, since she knew she was a squirter. Although, she had prefaced ahead of time that she doesn't always squirt. So, I guess I was just lucky or maybe we bi-women know a few tricks.

In the meantime, the trio up on the bed were into some serious sex. Mr. Hawaiian had Ms. Biceps mounted from behind while her boyfriend was lying on his back in front of her and she was sucking his unit quite enthusiastically. I went over just to play with her nipples, while my husband was still busy with the other lady. I heard Ms. Micro Mini, say to my husband while smacking her lips, "Did you recently have a condom on because I'm allergic to condoms." When I heard that a red flag immediately went up. She is allergic to condoms? She had already stated a couple times during the play that she wanted to be fucked by my husband. What was she thinking? We had stated in our profile, "Condoms Only". At this point, I couldn't figure out what she had on her mind so I just disappeared into the bathroom. When I came back to my husband, he immediately asked me if I was ready to leave. Since I was less than enthusiastic about the men and Ms Biceps was busy, we decided to end the evening early. We thanked all of them for our fun and as I got dressed, Mr. Hawaiian said that his girlfriend would help us out and unlock the padlock to the gate. Ms. Micro Mini had disappeared while I was in the bathroom. Nevertheless, we finished dressing and went to stand outside by the gate. We waited and waited and waited. Finally my husband said, "Screw it….let me help you climb over the wall." I told him to go ahead and pull the car around and I'd wait for the gate to open. He scaled over the 10 foot concrete wall and pulled the car around. She finally shows up fully clothed and unlocks the pad lock and I thanked her for her hospitality and climbed into the car with a huge grin on my face. My husband and I both burst out laughing at the same time. We must have talked about that evening for days. Obviously, this was *not* a typical swing date for us and we found humor and fun in it and just enjoyed it for what it was to us. It was entertainment value and nothing else. I enjoyed the evening with my husband and we shared laughs together. We had some fun with others, but it wasn't one at the top of our list for sexual excitement, but nonetheless was entertaining by its own merits. I mean, come on, I saw my first female squirter. As with anything in life, what do you do when you get lemons? You get your juicer out! Realties in life do not change, only your perspective. If you don't like something then change your perspective. It's that simple.

This line of thinking is also good when remembering the "doing one for the team" situations. I don't recommend anyone getting into a situation that both partners aren't 100% in agreement. Having fun with my husband has always been more important than the side issues of the actual sexual play experiences themselves. If you can't have fun with a given situation then step back and pull your partner aside and tell them you just can't do one for the team. Sometimes there will be no escaping that feeling and it's best just to pass and move on. Everyone has their limits and they are unique for each person.

Try not to allow the few bad experiences you may encounter outweigh your wonderful experiences. There will be plenty of positive experiences with others, so don't allow it to discourage you. Take the bad and gain insight and knowledge and relish in the positive experiences.

Remember, no one in life can make you happy or make you fulfilled. This can only come from within yourself. This is why too many people entering the Lifestyle with unhappiness find that participating in the Lifestyle doesn't make them happier. The Lifestyle, as with anything else in life, is what you make of it. Take as little or as much as you like and fit it to meet your needs, desires and standards. There are no right or wrong ways to playing with other people. You decide what is best for the two of you and have fun with it. There will be times when you need a break and will go for months with not much thought about it or any interest. Other times, your cup will be running over and the two of you can't get enough. Go out and have fun and enjoy each other.....with others. The most enjoyable part of a swing date for me is going home and snuggling up to my husband and making love. Embraced in his arms with the titillations of the evenings previous events, makes for powerful intimacy between us. There is nothing that can match the intimacy of your loved one. Everything else is just icing on the cake.

RESOURCES

There are hundreds of internet websites for swinging. Many are great and some offer free membership. Here are few sites that will get you started in the Lifestyle.

Websites

www.swinglifestyle.com

www.couples2couples.com

www.theswingsite.com

www.sdc.com

Club Forums
http://groups.yahoo.com/group/EliteSwingersofSoCal/

Sensual Accessories
www.amorouslinens.com

Made in the USA